Neuroanatomy
Made Easy
and
Understandable

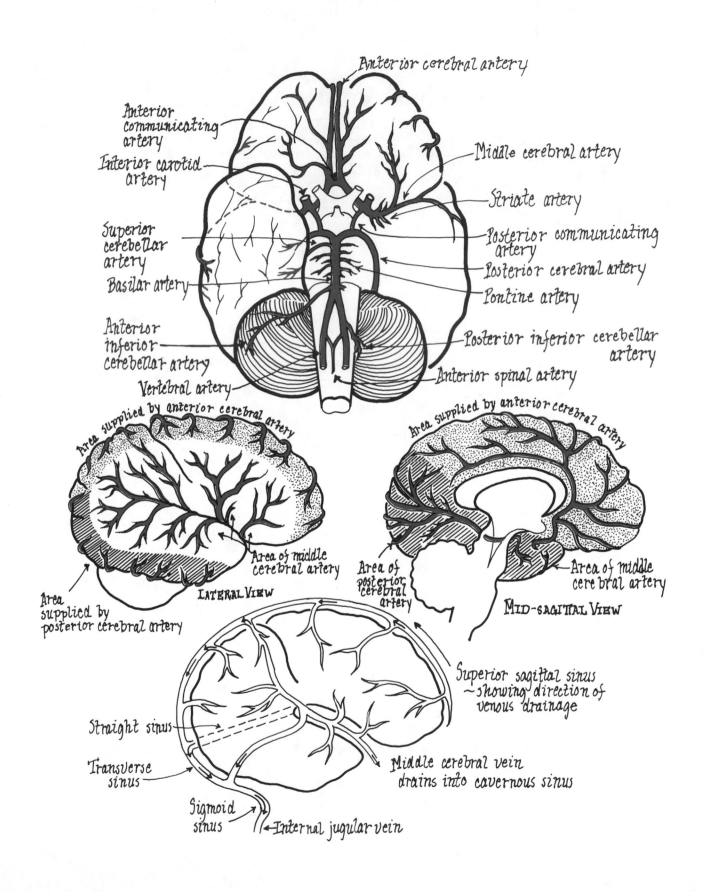

Anterior cerebral artery

Anterior communicating artery

Interior carotid artery

Superior cerebellar artery

Basilar artery

Anterior inferior cerebellar artery

Vertebral artery

Middle cerebral artery

Striate artery

Posterior communicating artery

Posterior cerebral artery

Pontine artery

Posterior inferior cerebellar artery

Anterior spinal artery

Area supplied by anterior cerebral artery

Area supplied by posterior cerebral artery

Area of middle cerebral artery

LATERAL VIEW

Area supplied by anterior cerebral artery

Area of posterior cerebral artery

Area of middle cerebral artery

MID-SAGITTAL VIEW

Superior sagittal sinus ~ showing direction of venous drainage

Straight sinus

Transverse sinus

Sigmoid sinus

Internal jugular vein

Middle cerebral vein drains into cavernous sinus

Neuroanatomy
Made Easy
and
Understandable

by

Michael Liebman, Ph.D.
Hadassah Medical School
The Hebrew University
Jerusalem

Visiting Lecturer
Department of Anatomy
Sackler School of Medicine
Tel-Aviv University

Visiting Lecturer
Ben Gurion University of the
Negev, Beersheba

and

former Professorial Lecturer in Anatomy
Department of Anatomy
The George Washington University Medical School
Washington, D.C.

University Park Press
Baltimore

UNIVERSITY PARK PRESS
International Publishers in Science, Medicine, and Education
300 North Charles Street
Baltimore, Maryland 21201

Composed by University Park Press, Typesetting Division.
Manufactured in the United States of America by
The Maple Press Company.
Second printing, March 1981
Third printing, October 1981

Library of Congress Cataloging Publication Data
Liebman, Michael.
Neuroanatomy made easy and understandable.

Bibliography: p.
Includes index.
1. Neuroanatomy. I. Title.
QM451.L53   611′.8   79-16292
ISBN 0-8391-1513-X

Contents

Don't Skip This Introduction

Today you are faced with the problem of having to know more and more material in a shorter and shorter period of time. With neuroanatomy this problem is compounded because it is one of the most difficult subjects to grasp. Most "neuro" texts are very broad in scope and crammed with details, the latest theories, and so on. At this stage, however, you're unable to "separate the wheat from the chaff," that is, to distinguish what is important for you from what is not. Consequently, you usually try to learn it all because you are afraid something will appear on the exam that you didn't "read up on." Under conditions of high pressure and little time, this usually results in a monumental effort of memory, accompanied by little understanding and retention.

In this book I have "cut out the fat" of extraneous details, theories, and the like, and left *the essentials that form the basis for neuroanatomy, neurophysiology, neuropharmacology, physical diagnosis, and neurology, and for passing exams.* Although the subject is presented in a deceptively simple, breezy, and personal style, you must not assume that it was done by sacrificing material. The main reason for this approach was to make the subject easier to read, understand, and retain. Therefore, once you know the material in this book, you will be able to read and quickly understand more detailed neuroanatomy texts and reference books, should the need arise.

The terminology can "throw you" for two reasons. First, it is often redundant. For example, a group of nerve fibers may be called a tract, fasciculus, column, lemniscus, funiculus, or bundle — all terms accepted and used by the medical and scientific community. Second, the terminology is full of weird sounding names of Greek and Latin origins. As for the first, the author obviously cannot at his whim cut out recognized terms, but he can point out those that are synonymous. As for the second problem, I have prepared a special glossary that not only explains the meaning and origin of the names but also lists a common everyday word derived from them. For example, *fornix* is a Latin word meaning an arch and is applied to a curved bundle of nerve fibers. The related everyday word is fornication, and the reason for this is that in ancient Rome the prostitutes used to hang around the arches of the aqueducts!

I strongly recommend that you read each chapter before going to each lecture; then, instead of furiously trying to write down every word, you'll be able to sit back, absorb, and understand the material and leisurely jot down additional notes and drawings.

Finally, I would welcome and appreciate suggestions and criticisms.

Good Luck!

*This book is dedicated
to my parents and
teachers*

Chapter 1

THE MICROSCOPIC BASIS OF NEUROANATOMY

The basic unit of the nervous system, as in all other systems of the body, is the cell, which here is called the *neuron.* The main properties that distinguish neurons from other types of cells are: their specialization for conduction of impulses, their great sensitivity to oxygen deprivation, their importance for many vital functions, and the fact that they don't multiply. (It is this last fact that is responsible for so many of the incurable conditions that you'll see — paralysis, chronic vegetative states, palsy, blindness, etc.) In this text we discuss many types of neurons, and they all have the above-mentioned characteristics.

A typical neuron (Figure 1) consists of a cell body with a large nucleus that has a dark, central *nucleolus.* Fine particles, known as *Nissl granules,* are scattered throughout most of the cytoplasm. Projecting from the cell body are many short processes, the *dendrites,* which receive impulses from other neurons and conduct them to the cell body. From the cell body a single long process, the *axon,* conducts the nerve impulse away and out to the dendrites of other neurons and to muscles and glands. The site of contact between the axon of one neuron and the dendrites of another is the *synapse,* but the impulse doesn't pass directly from neuron to neuron. Rather, it is transmitted by a chemical mediator known as *acetylcholine* and the basic mechanism is as follows: the nervous impulse, which is measurable with fine instruments, travels down the axon until it reaches the synapse. Here it causes the release of acetylcholine from the end of the axon and this passes through the ultra-microscopic synapseal gap to the adjacent dendrites, where it triggers a new impulse that is then propagated in the second neuron (Figure 1).

The axons of nearly all neurons are covered with a fatty white substance called *myelin;* in order for most impulses to be propagated, it must be present. In infants myelin hasn't been laid down completely and therefore they are unable to walk, while in certain diseases, such as multiple sclerosis, the myelin degenerates and the patient suffers from a loss of various sensations and/or a diminution of movements. The process of *myelinization* (laying down of myelin) is performed by special cells that form an outer enveloping layer around the axon known as the *sheath of Schwann (neurolemma).* Myelin is not a continuous layer but has gaps — the *nodes of Ranvier* — and here the overlying sheath of Schwann dips down and comes in contact with the axon (Figure 1).

Functionally and structurally there are many kinds of neurons; several of the most common are shown in Figure 2. A *motor* or *efferent neuron* is one that transmits impulses to muscles and/or glands, while a *sensory* or *afferent neuron* propagates sensory impulses. The nervous tissue of the brain and spinal cord is divided into *gray matter,* which is composed of the nerve cell bodies, and the *white matter,* which is made up of the white axon fibers. Furthermore, it has special cells — the *glia* — which are divided into three types: the first are *astrocytes,* whose functions are to hold together the delicate neurons and to create the blood-brain barrier that prevents many substances from leaving the capillaries to enter the brain tissue; the second are the *microglia,* which act as scavengers (*phagocytes*); and the last are the *oligodendroglia.* (The astrocytes and oligodendroglia are the macrophages.) Since the axons within the spinal cord and brain don't have a sheath of Schwann, it's thought that the oligodendroglia in these

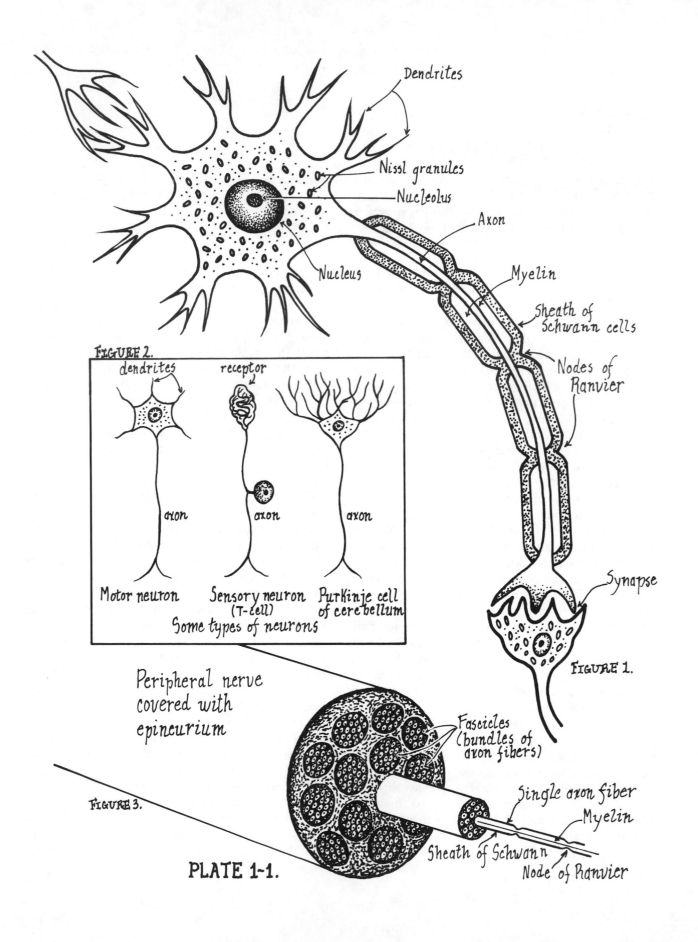

Dendrites

Nissl granules

Nucleolus

Axon

Myelin

Sheath of
Schwann cells

Nodes of
Ranvier

Nucleus

Synapse

FIGURE 1.

FIGURE 2.

dendrites

receptor

axon

axon

axon

Motor neuron

Sensory neuron
(T-cell)

Purkinje cell
of cerebellum

Some types of neurons

Peripheral nerve
covered with
epineurium

Fascicles
(bundles of
axon fibers)

Single axon fiber

Myelin

Sheath of Schwann

Node of Ranvier

FIGURE 3.

PLATE 1-1.

areas lay down the myelin. In addition to neurons and glia there are the *ependymal cells* that line the central canal, the *ventricles,* and which were the first cells to appear during the embryonic development of the nervous system.

Although the nerve pathways in the figures in other chapters are represented by a single axon, this is artistic license for the sake of clarity. In reality every nerve and pathway is made up of many bundles, called *fascicles,* which in turn are made up of hundreds and hundreds of axons (Figure 3).

CLINICAL ASPECTS

Since mature neurons don't multiply they are unable to give rise to brain tumors. The great majority of *neoplasms,* i.e., *tumors,* arise from glial cells or from the proliferation of other tissue cells found in conjunction with the brain, such as connective tissue or the epithelial cells of the pituitary gland, etc. Very rarely, neurons still in an immature state will give rise to tumors known as *neuroblastomas.*

When a nerve is cut, a series of characteristic reactions takes place. That part of the axon distal to the injury quickly breaks down and dies, a process known as *Wallerian degeneration.* The section of axon still attached to the cell body initially undergoes some degeneration, but if the damage isn't too extensive, it'll start growing. However, its growth is inhibited by the rapid proliferation of Schwann cells, which form a dense, scar-like mass. In cases where the severed ends of a nerve are sewn back together, growth will occur and there'll be some renewal of normal function. The amount of renewal depends on such factors as the degree of injury, the quickness and skill of repair, and the amount of glial cell proliferation at the repaired site.

Chapter 2

THE MACROSCOPIC BASIS OF NEUROANATOMY

This chapter deals with the macroscopic, many-named areas of the brain and is very boring. However, it is necessary because one can't proceed with the study of nervous pathways without knowing where they start, through what structures they pass, and where they end.

The nervous system is divided arbitrarily into a central and a peripheral part. The *central nervous system* (CNS) includes the *brain*, with its 12 pairs of *cranial nerves*, and the *spinal cord*, with 31 pairs of attached *spinal nerves*. The *peripheral nervous system* is made up of all the remaining nerves of the body and their associated collections of cell bodies — the *ganglia* — and is seen in the gross dissection of the cadaver.

FIVE PARTS OF THE BRAIN

The brain is divided on an embryological basis into five parts: *telencephalon, diencephalon, mesencephalon, pons* and *cerebellum*, and the *medulla oblongata*. In this chapter we consider these five parts one by one. The telencephalon is the center for the highest functions and is therefore the most developed in man. It is composed of two major structures: the *cerebral hemispheres* and the *basal ganglia*. The latter — areas for crude motor activity — are buried deep in the cerebral hemispheres and can only be seen when the brain is cut. The cerebral hemispheres, on the other hand, are two very large structures divided from each other by the *median longitudinal fissure* and comprise most of the brain matter that is seen (Figure 1).

Their convex surface is made up of convolutions called *gyri*, which are separated from each other by shallow grooves, the *sulci* (a deep sulcus is called a fissure). Two grooves, the lateral *fissure* and the *central sulcus*, help divide each hemisphere into four main areas, or *lobes* (Figure 2). The *frontal lobe* is anterior to the central sulcus and the *parietal lobe* is posterior to it (Figure 2). Lying below the *lateral fissure* is the *temporal lobe*, while an imaginary line drawn down from the *parieto-occipital fissure* separates the parietal lobe from the *occipital lobe* (Figure 2). As if there weren't enough divisions, each lobe has its specific areas and gyri. For example, in the frontal lobe the *precentral gyrus*, lying just anterior to the central sulcus, is the motor center that initiates impulses to the voluntary muscles. The most anterior area, the *frontal pole*, is the seat of personality (Figure 3), and injuries here often result in alterations of personality. These and other areas are discussed later in greater detail.

Telencephalon

The telencephalon also occupies much of the base of the brain. Here are situated the *orbital gyri* and resting on them are found the *olfactory nerve* and the *optic nerve*, which transmits visual impulses from the eye to the brain (Figure 4). The optic nerves converge on each other, cross at the *chiasma*, and then proceed posteriorly as the *optic tracts* (Figure 4). This view of the telencephalon also reveals the *hippocampal gyrus* of the temporal pole with its characteristic bulge, the *uncus*.

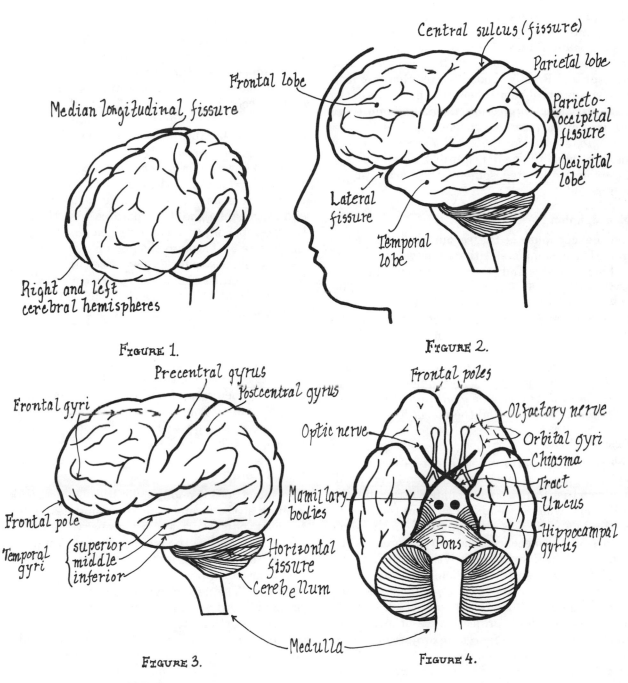

Median longitudinal fissure

Right and left cerebral hemispheres

FIGURE 1.

Central sulcus (fissure)

Frontal lobe

Parietal lobe

Parieto-occipital fissure

Occipital lobe

Lateral fissure

Temporal lobe

FIGURE 2.

Frontal gyri

Precentral gyrus

Postcentral gyrus

Frontal pole

Temporal gyri

{ superior middle inferior

Horizontal fissure

Cerebellum

Medulla

FIGURE 3.

Frontal poles

Optic nerve

Mamillary bodies

Pons

Olfactory nerve

Orbital gyri

Chiasma

Tract

Uncus

Hippocampal gyrus

FIGURE 4.

PLATE 2~1.

When the brain is cut in a horizontal plane, one sees that the cerebral hemispheres have an outer gray layer, the *cortex,* which is composed of cell bodies, and an inner white mass made up of myelinated axons (Figure 5). Axons that pass from one hemisphere to the other are called *commissural fibers,* and the best example of this is the large *corpus callosum* (Figures 5 and 6). *Associative fibers* are those that pass from lobe to lobe in the same hemisphere. Finally, those axons that descend from the cerebral hemisphere to other areas of the CNS are called *projection fibers* and most are situated in the *internal capsule.* This has an *anterior limb,* a *posterior limb,* and a section between the two called the *genu* (Figure 5). Just lateral to the genu are located some of the basal ganglia (Figure 5).

Diencephalon

The diencephalon is the second division of the brain. It is a small area situated between the cerebral hemispheres and is seen best on a mid-sagittal view (Figure 6). The diencephalon is divided into the *thalamus,* which is the main relay center for the nervous system, and, below it, the *hypothalamus* (Figure 6). The hypothalamus is a vital area concerned with temperature control, emotional states, and control over the autonomic nervous system. In addition, the diencephalon is made up of the *medial* and *lateral geniculate bodies,* the *subthalamic nucleus,* and the *pineal body.*

Mesencephalon

The remaining parts of the brain — the mesencephalon, the pons and cerebellum, and the medulla — together form a wedge-shaped structure, the *brainstem,* which extends down from the base of the brain to the *foramen magnum* of the skull (Figure 6). The mesencephalon, or *midbrain,* is the smallest of the five divisions of the brain and is located between the diencephalon and the pons (Figure 6). The area above the *aqueduct of Sylvius* (cerebral aqueduct) is the *tectum,* which is made up of four rounded projections — the *corpora quadrigemina.* The upper two projections form the *superior colliculus* and the lower two, the *inferior colliculus.* In the body or *tegmentum* of the midbrain pass various fiber tracts. Also situated there are: the *red nucleus* and the *substantia nigra,* the *oculomotor nerve* and its nucleus, and the *trochlear nerve* and its nucleus. Finally, at the base of the midbrain there is a pair of huge fiber bundles, the *cerebral peduncles,* which are a con-

tinuation of the descending projection fibers of the internal capsule (Figure 6a). (The cerebral peduncles are also called *crus cerebri* or the *basis pedunculi.)*

Pons and Cerebullum

The pons and cerebellum make up the fourth division of the brain (Figure 6). The cerebellum is a many-folded structure under the occipital lobe and is concerned with equilibrium, muscle tone, and the coordination of muscle activity. Passing between it and the underlying brainstem are three pairs of fiber bundles: the *superior, middle,* and *inferior cerebellar peduncles* (see Chapter 11). They are also known as the *brachium conjunctivum,* the *brachium pontis,* and the *restiform body,* respectively. The pons is located between the midbrain and the medulla and it's separated from the overlying cerebellum by a cavity — the *fourth ventricle* (Figure 6). Through the pons pass various ascending and descending fiber tracts. It is also the locus of the fifth cranial nerve (*trigeminal nerve*), the sixth cranial nerve (*abducens*), and the seventh cranial nerve (the *facial nerve*).

Medulla Oblongata

The medulla oblongata is the last division of the brain. It becomes continuous with the spinal cord at the foramen magnum (Figure 6). Like the pons and midbrain it contains ascending and descending fiber tracts, as well as the nuclei of cranial nerves VIII through XII.

Spinal Cord

The spinal cord is a long cylindrical structure beginning at the foramen magnum and descending to about the level of the third lumbar vertebra (L_3). The cord serves as the main pathway — highway — for the ascending and descending fiber tracts that connect the peripheral and spinal nerves with the brain. The peripheral nerves are attached to the spinal cord by 31 pairs of spinal nerves.

A cross-section of the spinal cord reveals gray matter in the form of an H or butterfly surrounded on all sides by white matter. As in the cerebral hemispheres, the gray matter is composed of cell bodies, while the white is the myelinated axon fibers (Figure 7). The upper limbs of the gray are the *dorsal* or *posterior horns,* while the lower are the *ventral* or *anterior horns.* The white matter is grouped into dorsal, ventral, and lateral *columns* (Figure 7).

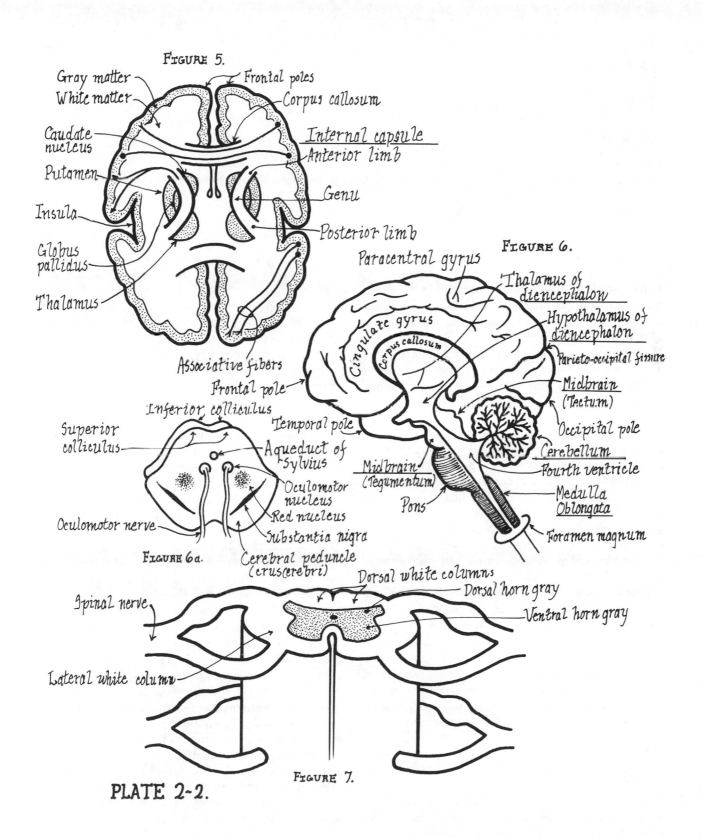

FIGURE 5.

Gray matter
White matter
Frontal poles
Corpus callosum
Caudate nucleus
Internal capsule
Anterior limb
Putamen
Genu
Insula
Posterior limb
Globus pallidus
Thalamus
Associative fibers
Frontal pole

FIGURE 6.

Paracentral gyrus
Thalamus of diencephalon
Cingulate gyrus
Corpus callosum
Hypothalamus of diencephalon
Parieto-occipital fissure
Midbrain (Tectum)
Occipital pole
Cerebellum
Fourth ventricle
Midbrain (Tegumentum)
Pons
Medulla Oblongata
Temporal pole
Foramen magnum

Inferior colliculus
Superior colliculus
Aqueduct of Sylvius
Oculomotor nucleus
Red nucleus
Oculomotor nerve
Substantia nigra
FIGURE 6a.
Cerebral peduncle (cruscerebri)

Dorsal white columns
Dorsal horn gray
Spinal nerve
Ventral horn gray
Lateral white column

FIGURE 7.

PLATE 2-2.

Chapter **3**

PAIN AND TEMPERATURE PATHWAY FROM THE EXTREMITIES AND TRUNK

Most people who consult a doctor do so because they are in pain. Therefore, a fundamental understanding of the pain and temperature pathway is essential to quick and accurate diagnosis. Fortunately, this is a simple pathway and a good grasp of it is easily obtained.

The receptors of pain and temperature are found in the dermis and epidermis of the skin. Nerve fibers pass from the dermis toward the spinal cord, with the cell bodies being situated in the dorsal root ganglion (Figure 1). The fibers then enter the cord through the dorsal root of the spinal nerve and end in the dorsal horn of the gray matter. Here the first neuron synapses with a second that then crosses to the contralateral (other) side of the cord, enters the lateral white column, and ascends to the ventral posterolateral nucleus of the thalamus (Figure 1). This ascending bundle of crossed pain and temperature fibers is known as the *lateral spinothalamic tract*. In the ventral posterolateral nucleus the axons of the lateral spinothalamic tract synapse with tertiary neurons that leave the thalamus and ascend in the internal capsule to reach the *postcentral gyrus* (Figure 1). The cortical gray matter of the postcentral gyrus (also known as area 3,1,2) is the primary somatic sensory area of the brain and is concerned with interpreting pain and temperature sensations, as well as other cutaneous sensations, such as pressure and touch (see following chapters).

ACCESSORY DETAILS

The primary pain and temperature axons have branches that synapse in the dorsal horn with short neurons that pass down to the ventral horn (Figure 1). Here these short *internuncial* (messenger) neurons synapse with motor neurons whose axons pass out through the ventral root and go out to voluntary muscles, causing movement. This involuntary motor response to a sensory stimulus is called a *reflex* and is a defense mechanism of the nervous system that permits quick, automatic responses to painful and potentially damaging situations. The internuncials may cross over to the other side of the cord and stimulate motor neurons there, or they may descend or ascend the cord and stimulate motor neurons at different levels of the cord. It all depends on the group of muscles that need to be "called into action."

The dorsal root of the spinal nerve is composed only of sensory (afferent) axons whose cell bodies are situated in the dorsal root ganglion. The ventral root, on the other hand, is made up exclusively of motor or efferent axons whose cell bodies are located in the gray matter of the ventral horn.

The fibers of each dorsal root come from a fairly circumscribed area of skin known as a *dermatome*. There is, however, at each boundary of the dermatome an area that is supplied by the adjacent segmental nerves and this overlap acts as a kind of biologic "insurance." For example, if the second thoracic nerve (T_2) is severed, then many of the pain and temperature sensations from the skin area supplied by T_2 will be carried by the T_1 and T_3 sensory neurons (Figure 2). There is also an overlap pattern in the spinal cord. The entering axon, before it passes into the dorsal horn, sends branches that ascend and descend one spinal segment in the dorsolateral fasciculus (or column) of Lissauer and then enter the dorsal horn at that segment (Figure 2).

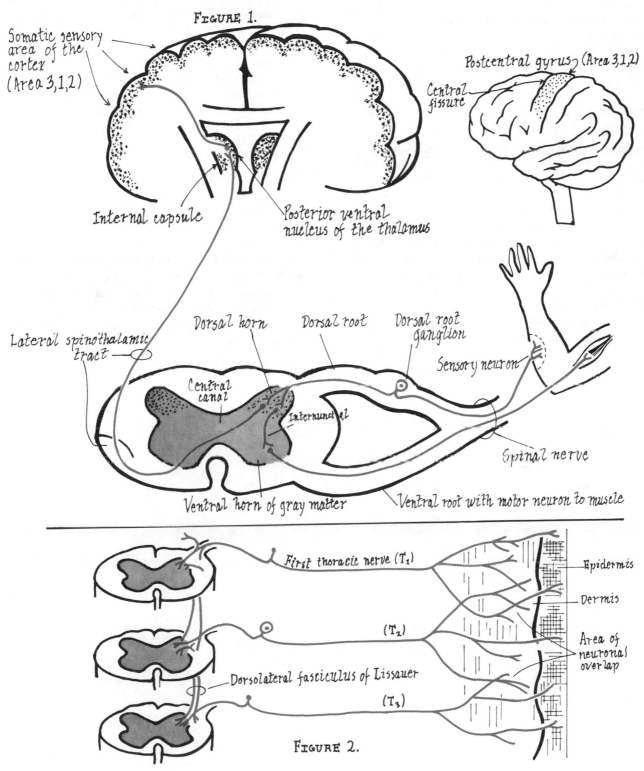

FIGURE 1.

Somatic sensory area of the cortex (Area 3,1,2)

Postcentral gyrus (Area 3,1,2)

Central fissure

Internal capsule

Posterior ventral nucleus of the thalamus

Dorsal horn   Dorsal root   Dorsal root ganglion

Lateral spinothalamic tract

Sensory neuron

Central canal

Internuncial

Spinal nerve

Ventral horn of gray matter

Ventral root with motor neuron to muscle

First thoracic nerve (T₁)

Epidermis

(T₂)

Dermis

Area of neuronal overlap

Dorsolateral fasciculus of Lissauer

(T₃)

FIGURE 2.

PLATE 3~1.

CLINICAL ASPECTS

Referred Pain

The pain and pathway from the viscera (internal organs) are poorly understood. Visceral pain is not well localized; in certain cases it isn't felt at the organ site, but is experienced at the surface of the body some distance from the affected organ. Such a reaction is known as referred pain and in many instances it is quite specific and can serve as an excellent diagnostic aid. For example: A person suffering from a coronary attack often experiences a sharp pain that radiates along the inner aspect of the left arm; pain originating from the ureters is felt in the testes; while pain from the lungs and diaphragm is experienced at the shoulders near the root of the neck. [An excellent discussion of the theories of referred pain is presented in Crosby's *Correlative Anatomy of the Nervous System,* page 83 (Macmillan, 1962).]

Phantom Limb

In many cases following amputation the patient complains to the doctor of excruciating pain from the fingers or toes that no longer exist!! The explanation for this strange phenomenon is as follows: A stimulus applied anywhere along the nerve fiber is experienced by the sensory cortex as coming not from the site of stimulation but rather from the skin area supplied by the nerves being stimulated. The nerve fibers at the stump are frequently squeezed by the scar tissue and this pain stimulus passes to the sensory cortex, which interprets it as coming not from the stump area but from the skin areas of the fingers or toes of the missing limb.

Cordotomy

In cases of severe pain, as, for example, from cancer, where drugs no longer alleviate the pain, a surgical procedure known as *cordotomy* is performed. The surgeon cuts the lateral spinothalamic tract of the cord, on the opposite side from the site of the pain and at a level one or two segments higher than the entrance of the uppermost spinal nerve that serves the affected area. The latter is done because of the overlap that exists in the cord (see above).

Chapter 4

PATHWAY FOR PRESSURE AND CRUDE TOUCH FROM THE EXTREMITIES AND TRUNK

The receptors for pressure and crude touch are situated in the dermis of the skin. The nerve fibers travel in the peripheral nerves toward the spinal cord. The cell bodies are aggregated in the dorsal root ganglion and from here axons enter the cord through the dorsal root (Figure 1). Upon entering, the axons pass into the ipsilateral (i.e., the same side) dorsal white column and bifurcate. One branch immediately enters the dorsal horn gray and synapses with a 2° neuron. The other branch ascends in the ipsilateral dorsal column for as many as ten spinal segments and then enters the dorsal horn gray to synapse with a 2° neuron (Figure 1). In both cases, the 2° neurons decussate, i.e., cross over to the other side, and enter the ventral white column, where they form the ventral spinothalamic tract. This tract ascends to the ventral posterolateral nucleus of the thalamus, where it synapses with 3° neurons (Figure 1), which then relay the pressure and crude touch sensations to the postcentral gyrus of the cortex, which is concerned with interpreting sensations.

CLINICAL ASPECTS

Because one branch of the 1° neuron synapses immediately with a 2° neuron, while the second branch ascends ipsilaterally for many segments, injuries to the spinal cord rarely result in complete loss of pressure and crude touch sensations. For example, if there is any injury to the spinal cord at point A in Figure 1 and the ventral spinothalamic tract is cut, one sees that the long ascending branch of the primary neuron bypasses the injury (on the uninjured side) and thus the sensations can still reach the postcentral gyrus. Naturally, if the sensory cortex, the internal capsule, or the thalamus is injured, then the pressure and crude touch sensations are lost on the opposite, or contralateral, side of the body.

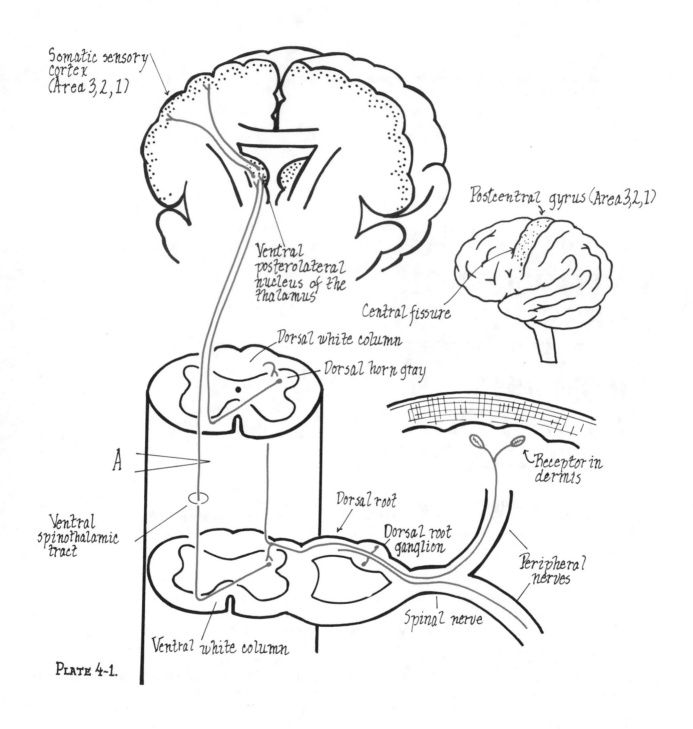

Somatic sensory cortex (Area 3, 2, 1)

Ventral posterolateral nucleus of the thalamus

Postcentral gyrus (Area 3, 2, 1)

Central fissure

Dorsal white column

Dorsal horn gray

A

Receptor in dermis

Ventral spinothalamic tract

Dorsal root

Dorsal root ganglion

Peripheral nerves

Spinal nerve

Ventral white column

Plate 4-1.

Chapter **5**

PATHWAY FOR PROPRIOCEPTION, FINE TOUCH, AND VIBRATORY SENSE FROM THE EXTREMITIES AND TRUNK

Three different sensations — proprioception, fine touch, and vibratory senses — all use the same pathway. *Proprioception* is the sense that enables one to know exactly and at all times where the parts of the body are, in space and in relation to each other. Thus, it enables a person, with the eyes closed, to bring up the hand and with the index finger to touch the tip of the nose. Its receptors are located in muscles, tendons, and joints. *Fine touch* is the sense that enables a person, again with the eyes closed, to identify various objects, such as keys, coins, ping-pong ball, etc., by touch, a property known in medicine as *stereognosis*. Fine touch also involves the facility to discriminate between two points when one is being touched by both points simultaneously, as with the two points of a compass. These receptors are situated in the dermis of the skin; and they are most sensitive in the fingertips and lips and least sensitive on the back. *Vibratory sense* is, as its name implies, the sensation of vibrating objects.

The fibers of all three sensations pass toward the spinal cord in the peripheral nerves, and the cell bodies are aggregated in the dorsal root ganglion. From here, axons enter the spinal cord and immediately pass into the ipsilateral dorsal white columns, where they ascend all the way up to the medulla (Figure 1). Axons that enter the cord at the sacral and lumbar levels are situated in the medial part of the dorsal column, which is called the *fasciculus gracilis*, while those axons that enter at the thoracic and cervical levels form the more lateral *fasciculus cuneatus* (Figure 1). The axons of each fasciculus terminate in their respective nucleus in the medulla. The 2° neurons leave the nucleus gracilis and cuneatus and cross over to the other side of the medulla, where they form a bundle known as the *medial lemniscus,* which ascends to the ventral posterolateral nucleus of the thalamus (Figure 1). Here the 2° neurons synapse with 3° neurons that pass up through the internal capsule to reach the postcentral gyrus, area 3,1,2, which is the primary cerebral somesthetic region.

CLINICAL ASPECTS

Damage to the postcentral gyrus, to the medial lemniscus, to the dorsal column, or to the cell

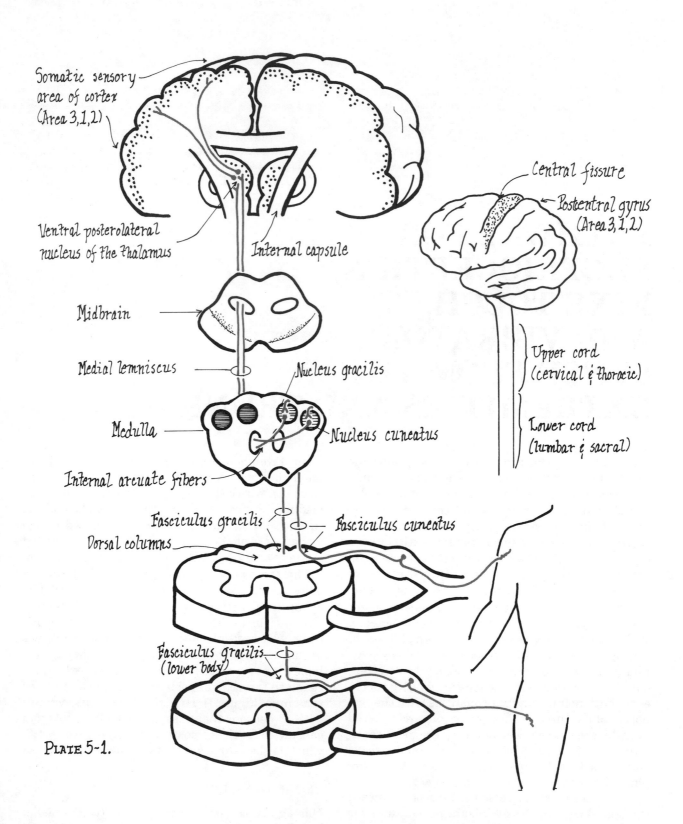

Somatic sensory
area of cortex
(Area 3,1,2)

Ventral posterolateral
nucleus of the thalamus

Internal capsule

Central fissure

Postcentral gyrus
(Area 3,1,2)

Midbrain

Medial lemniscus

Nucleus gracilis

Medulla

Nucleus cuneatus

Internal arcuate fibers

Upper cord
(cervical & thoracic)

Lower cord
(lumbar & sacral)

Fasciculus gracilis

Fasciculus cuneatus

Dorsal columns

Fasciculus gracilis
(lower body)

PLATE 5-1.

bodies in the dorsal root ganglion* results in several distinct clinical symptoms:

1. Astereognosis — loss of ability to distinguish between objects through touch and manipulation.
2. Loss of vibratory sense.
3. Loss of two-point tactile discrimination — when touched simultaneously with two points of a compass, the patient says he feels one.
4. A loss of proprioception, so that there's an inability to know where the limbs are. There-

---

*This occurs in the third stage of syphilis, when the organisms selectively attack and destroy these cell bodies but initially spare those of pain, temperature, crude touch, and pressure.

fore, such a patient looks down at his feet when walking, and at night would stagger or fall. When he is asked to stand erect with both feet together and eyes closed, his body sways — a positive Romberg sign.

If the injury is bilateral, then, of course, the symptoms will be on both sides of the body. If, however, the lesion is on one side, then the symptoms will appear on one side only, depending on where the damage is. If the damage is before the decussation, i.e., the dorsal root ganglion, the posterior column, or medullary nuclei, then the signs will be on the same side; if it is after the decussation, i.e., the medial lemniscus, the thalamus, or cerebral cortex, then the signs will be on the side opposite to the lesion.

Chapter 6

SENSORY PATHWAYS FROM THE FACE AND RELATED AREAS

Our discussions of somatic sensory pathways don't include nerves from the face and related areas because these areas don't "use" the spinal nerves. Sensations for these areas pass in the fifth cranial nerve, the trigeminal. The basic groundplan is pretty much the same and an understanding of it is important, especially for those studying dentistry or those who have chosen a specialty involving the cranial region.

The trigeminal nerve is the major somatic sensory nerve for the face, the anterior half of the scalp, the mouth cavity, the meninges, the sinuses, the teeth, the tongue, the cornea, and the outer surface of the eardrum. It transmits the sensations of pain and temperature and all kinds of touch, pressure, and proprioception, but not those of the special senses, such as hearing, taste, smell, vision, and equilibrium, which are carried by other cranial nerves.

PAIN AND TEMPERATURE
PATHWAY (solid lines in Figure 1)

From receptors situated in the above-mentioned areas, fibers pass in the peripheral branches of the trigeminal nerve toward the brain. Their cell bodies are located in the *semilunar* or *Gasserian ganglion* (Figure 1), which is the analogue of the dorsal root ganglion. From here the axons enter the pons and are immediately concentrated in a bundle, the descending or spinal tract of V, which swings down and in many cases reaches the upper cervical region of the cord. Along this course the primary neurons peel off and enter the adjacent nucleus of the descending tract of V where they synapse with secondary neurons. These leave the nucleus, cross over to the contralateral side, and ascend to terminate in the ventral posteromedial nucleus of the thalamus (Figure 1). This crossed and ascending pain and temperature bundle is

called the ventral 2° ascending V and is analogous to the lateral spinothalamic tract. From the thalamus, tertiary neurons pass into the internal capsule, ascend in it, and end in the postcentral gyrus (area 3,1,2) — the somesthetic (somatic sensory) region of the cortex.

PRESSURE AND TOUCH
PATHWAY (dotted lines in Figure 1)

These neurons also have their cell bodies in the semilunar ganglion, but their axons terminate immediately in the main sensory nucleus of V situated in the pons (Figure 1). The secondary neurons reach the ventral posteromedial nucleus of the thalamus via the dorsal 2° ascending V, which is a crossed and uncrossed track, i.e., some axons travel ipsilaterally and some contralaterally and thus resemble the pressure and touch pathway for the body. Tertiary neurons are relayed from the thalamus to the postcentral gyrus (Figure 1). Thus, we see that, whereas pain and temperature are projected on the contralateral cerebral cortex, pressure and touch are bilaterally projected. Therefore, if one side of the sensory cortex is damaged, the patient will suffer no loss of pressure and touch from the face but he will lose the pain and temperature feelings on the contralateral side.

PROPRIOCEPTION PATHWAY (Figure 2)

There are trigemino-proprioceptive fibers from the muscles of mastication and from the temperomandibular joint. However, they are an exception in that their 1° cell bodies aren't in a ganglion outside the CNS but are situated in the mesencephalic nucleus in the midbrain. The further pathway of this sensation to the postcentral gyrus is not well known.

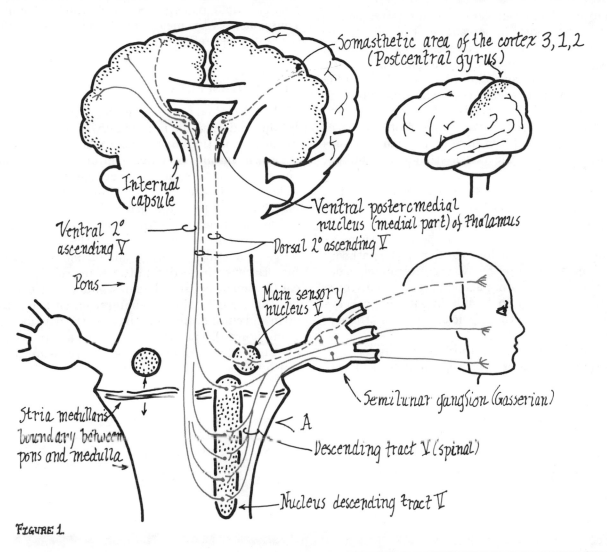

Somasthetic area of the cortex 3,1,2
(Postcentral gyrus)

Internal capsule

Ventral postero-medial
nucleus (medial part) of thalamus

Ventral 2° ascending V

Dorsal 2° ascending V

Pons →

Main sensory nucleus V

Semilunar ganglion (Gasserian)

Stria medullaris boundary between pons and medulla →

A

Descending tract V (spinal)

Nucleus descending tract V

FIGURE 1.

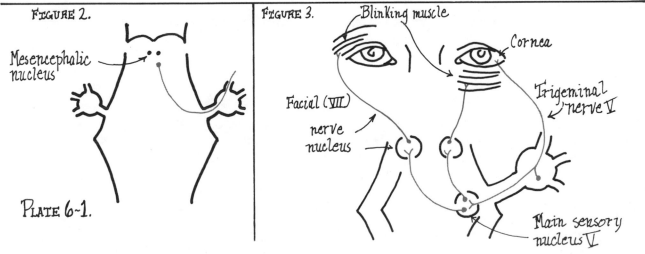

FIGURE 2.

Mesencephalic nucleus

PLATE 6-1.

FIGURE 3.

Blinking muscle

Cornea

Facial (VII)

Trigeminal nerve V

nerve nucleus

Main sensory nucleus V

ACCESSORY DETAIL

There are several reflexes involving the trigeminal nerve; the most important is the corneal or "blink" reflex. If an object touches the cornea of one eye, both of them will blink immediately. The pathway is as follows: the touch stimulus from the cornea reaches the ipsilateral main sensory nucleus V. This sends out internuncial neurons that pass to the *right and left* motor nuclei of the facial nerve. From here motor neurons pass out and stimulate the muscles that cause blinking (Figure 3).

Reflexes not only are a defense mechanism but also are useful diagnostically, enabling the doctor to test the integrity of nerve pathways. If, upon testing, a reflex is not elicited, the doctor then has to find out where the interruption in the pathway is: in the sensory pathway, the internuncial connections, or the motor pathway. In addition, there are reflexes that appear only in pathological conditions, informing the physician that something is wrong.

When a person is anesthetized in surgery, specific reflexes disappear as deeper and deeper levels of unconsciousness are reached. Thus, the anesthetist is able to gauge accurately the level of unconsciousness by means of the presence or absence of these reflexes.

CLINICAL ASPECTS

If the trigeminal nerve or the semilunar ganglion is damaged, then the individual will suffer loss of all facial sensations on the same side as the injury. As was mentioned previously, injury to one side of the sensory cortex, internal capsule, etc., results in loss of facial pain and temperature contralaterally, but pressure and touch will remain.

Trigeminal neuralgia (tic douloureux) is a condition of unknown etiology in which the patient suffers excruciating, shooting pain on one side of the face. Because drugs don't often bring relief, surgical treatment is used. The descending tract of V lies superficially, thus enabling neurosurgeons to go in and cut it on the side that has the pain (point A in Figure 1). Thus they sever the pain and temperature axons while sparing the pressure and touch fibers.

Chapter **7**

PATHWAY FOR VOLUNTARY MUSCLE ACTIVITY

Everyone has undoubtedly seen at one time or another individuals who can't walk and are confined to wheelchairs, or who walk slowly, dragging one leg, or whose arm lies helplessly at one side; in short, persons who have some form of paralysis. In all these conditions the muscles are fundamentally intact, and the condition is due to some kind of injury to the nerves. Since damage to no other pathway is responsible for so much suffering and sorrow, a first-class understanding of this pathway is mandatory.

The *corticospinal tract* is the main tract for nearly all voluntary muscle activity. It originates in the precentral gyrus (area 4, the motor cortex) of the frontal lobe. Here are located its large cell bodies, and since many of them have a pyramidal shape, the corticospinal tract is also called the *pyramidal tract.* (How a conscious wish is "translated" into cortical nerve impulses is an age-old question involving the mind-matter problem, and probably will never be answered satisfactorily.) From the cell bodies, axons leave the cortex and pass down through the internal capsule, which isn't a capsule, but the main passageway for ascending and descending fiber tracts (Figure 1). Leaving the internal capsule, the axon fibers pass down into the basis pedunculi of the midbrain and continue down the brainstem to reach the medulla oblongata. Here about 80–90% of the axons decussate to the opposite or contralateral side of the medulla and, having crossed over, descend in the spinal cord (Figure 1). Since these descending fibers are situated in the lateral white columns of the cord they are called the lateral corticospinal tract. Those axons that don't cross over in the medulla continue down on the same side to enter the ventral white columns of the spinal cord and are therefore known as the ventral corticospinal tract.

At each level of the cord, axons from the lateral corticospinal tract peel off and enter the gray matter of the ventral horn, where they terminate by synapsing with second-order neurons. At each corresponding level of the cord, axons of the ventral corticospinal tract peel off and cross over to the other side of the cord (Figure 1). Here they also enter and terminate upon 2° neurons in the ventral horn. It must be emphasized that, in their entire course from the precentral gyrus to the ventral horn, both the lateral and ventral corticospinal tracts consist of single uninterrupted neurons, i.e., the tracts are a single neuron pathway. These neurons are called *upper motor neurons.* The second-order neurons, on which the upper motor neurons synapse, send their axons out of the spinal cord via the ventral roots. They then branch out in the peripheral nerves and supply the voluntary muscles. These 2° neurons are *lower motor neurons,* and this differentiation between them and the upper motor neurons is very important clinically, as we shall soon see. In a person who is 6′ tall, the axons that supply the toe muscles are nearly a yard long. The upper motor neurons begin in the precentral gyrus and end in the lower part of the cord, while the lower motor neuron begins in the lower cord and its axon passes down to supply the muscle situated on the sole of the foot.

DETAILS

Cerebral Localization

The nerve cell bodies of the upper motor neurons are arranged in a specific pattern in the gray matter of the precentral gyrus so that neurons supplying the foot and leg muscles are situated dorsomedially in the gyrus. As one passes inferolaterally one finds the area for the abdomen, chest, arm, hand, and face. One can describe this more colorfully by saying that the pattern is that of a person hanging upside down, with the feet in the longitudinal fissure and the head at the edge of the lateral fissure (Figure 1). The area of neurons that supply muscles of the hand is disproportionately large,

19

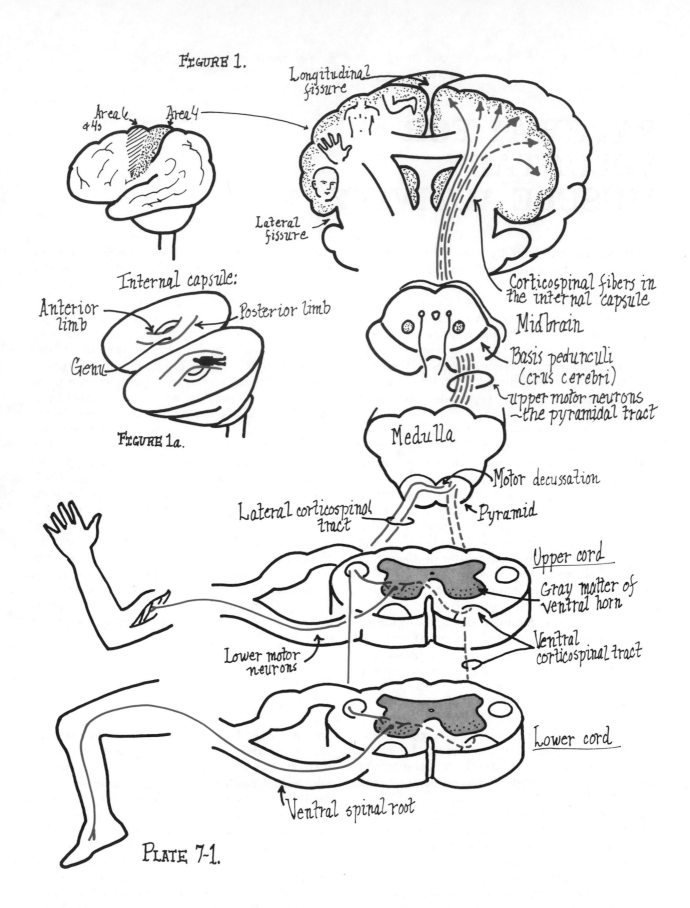

FIGURE 1.

Longitudinal fissure

Area 6 & 4s

Area 4

Lateral fissure

Internal capsule:

Anterior limb

Posterior limb

Genu

FIGURE 1a.

Corticospinal fibers in the internal capsule

Midbrain

Basis pedunculi (crus cerebri)

upper motor neurons ~ the pyramidal tract

Medulla

Motor decussation

Lateral corticospinal tract

Pyramid

Upper cord

Gray matter of ventral horn

Lower motor neurons

Ventral corticospinal tract

Lower cord

Ventral spinal root

PLATE 7-1.

reflecting the great number of neurons needed to carry out fine and complicated movements, such as violin playing, surgery, etc. This localization is also seen in the internal capsule, the main cerebral passageway for ascending and descending fiber tracts. In a horizontal section (Figure 1a) of the cerebral hemisphere one sees that the internal capsule consists of an anterior limb, a posterior limb, and a connecting area between them, the genu. The fibers that supply the face are situated in the genu, and those supplying the rest of the body are found in the anterior two-thirds of the posterior limb. If the genu is damaged, then the muscles of the face are affected, but if the middle part of the posterior limb is injured, then the leg muscles won't get nervous supply.

Suppressor Part of the Pyramidal Tract

Not all the neurons of the pyramidal tract have their origins in the precentral gyrus. Many of them originate in areas 4s and 6, which lie just anterior to the precentral gyrus (Figure 1). Pyramidal tract fibers originating here do not initiate impulses to voluntary muscles, but act as inhibitors, suppressors, or "brakes" on the lower motor neurons and prevent them from over-discharging when responding reflexively to sensory stimuli. If for some reason the suppressor fibers are damaged, then the lower motor neurons are freed from their control and "fire" excessively in response to reflex stimuli or discharge spontaneously. These conditions are known as *hyperreflexion* and *spasticity,* and are discussed in the next section.

CLINICAL ASPECTS

Lower Motor Neuron Paralysis

The best examples of lower motor neuron paralysis are: when a nerve to a muscle is cut or when the cell bodies of the ventral horn are destroyed by poliomyelitis virus, which selectively attacks them. In both cases the muscles are deprived of their immediate nerve supply; they are unable to contract and become soft, flabby, and atrophic — characteristics of a flaccid paralysis. Naturally, since the motor limb of the reflex arc is damaged, the muscles can't respond reflexively to sensory stimuli.

Upper Motor Neuron Paralysis

Upper motor neuron paralysis occurs when there is damage to the corticospinal tract anywhere along its path: the cell bodies in the precentral gyrus or their descending axons in the internal capsule, brainstem, or spinal cord. The most common site of injury is in the cerebral hemisphere, before the decussation. Injury results most often when an artery becomes stopped up and the neurons, deprived of their oxygen supply, die, producing what's known as a cerebrovascular accident (CVA) or, in popular language, a *stroke.* If the site affected is above the motor decussation, then the signs and symptoms will be seen in the muscles on the opposite side of the body. If the injury is after the decussation, say a cut in the left half of the spinal cord, then the ensuing paralysis will be on the same side as the damage. This type of paralysis is different from a lower motor neuron paralysis in a number of essential ways. First of all, the lower motor neurons are not affected and the reflex arc is complete, and thus reflexes can be elicited. Secondly, the suppressor fibers originating in areas 4s and 6 are knocked out and their braking effect on the lower motor neurons is no longer effective. The lower motor neurons now over-discharge to stimuli or even "fire" spontaneously. Clinically, this hyperreflexia manifests itself as follows: when the wrist of a paralyzed arm is grasped firmly, there will be a series of rapid, strong, muscular contractions, known as *clonus.* When the lower motor neurons discharge spontaneously, the muscles contract strongly, a condition known as spasticity. Thus, upper motor neuron paralysis is spastic, as opposed to lower motor neuron paralysis, which is flaccid. In upper motor neuron paralysis a characteristic and specific type of reflex — the Babinski reflex — can be elicited. When the sole of the foot of a healthy person is stroked in a heel-to-toe direction, the toes will curl. However, in a patient who has an upper motor neuron lesion, the toes will fan apart and the big toe will flex dorsally. The exact route and mechanism of the Babinski reflex are still not fully understood. (In a normal infant up to the age of six months or so, where the myelinization of the axons is not complete, a Babinski response can be elicited routinely.) Also, certain superficial reflexes, such as the abdominal and cremasteric, elicited when the skin is stroked, are lost. Once again the exact reason and mechanism are not clear.

A person who is "paralyzed" on one side of the body can frequently make crude movements of the trunk musculature on the affected side. The explanation for this is as follows: It is known that some of the ventral corticospinal fibers don't cross over at all, and it is believed that these uncrossed fibers, along with some of the crossed ones, supply the muscles of the trunk. Thus the trunk muscles of each side receive axons from both the right and left cerebral cortex. This arrangement is known as *bilateral innervation.*

Definitions: Monoplegia is paralysis of either an upper or a lower limb; hemiplegia is paralysis of an upper and a lower limb on the same side; paraplegia is paralysis of both lower limbs; quadriplegia is paralysis of all four limbs.

Chapter 8

PATHWAY TO VOLUNTARY MUSCLES OF THE HEAD

Our discussion of the pyramidal tract centered on those fibers that descend into the spinal cord and synapse there with lower motor neurons that go out and innervate voluntary muscles of the body. It didn't include fibers to the muscles of the head because the lower motor neurons supplying them aren't situated in spinal nerves but are associated with cranial nerves originating in the brainstem. The basic framework, however, is the same as for the corticospinal tracts. Namely, it is a two-neuron pathway consisting of an upper motor neuron originating in the cerebral cortex whose axon descends and synapses with a lower motor neuron that in turn goes out and stimulates voluntary muscles.

The cell bodies of the upper motor neurons are located in the lowest part of the precentral gyrus (motor cortex — area 4) adjacent to the lateral fissure (Figure 1). There is in addition another motor area for eyeball movements that is situated in the middle frontal gyrus (Figure 1a). Axons from here join descending fibers from the face area and together they pass through the genu of the internal capsule. Since the fibers then enter the brainstem or bulb, and terminate on lower motor neurons, they are called the *corticobulbar tract*, in contradistinction to the corticospinal tract. The cell bodies of the lower motor are concentrated in specific areas of the brainstem called *nuclei* and their axons form many of the cranial nerves. These nerves differ from spinal nerves in that the sensory and motor fibers don't separate into dorsal and ventral roots. Furthermore, some cranial nerves don't have any sensory axons but all their fibers are lower motor neurons. To complicate the matter even further, there are cranial nerves that are entirely sensory in their make-up. Be that as it may, the cranial nerves that interest us here are those whose axons supply voluntary muscles, and these are: the oculomotor (III) and the trochlear (IV) nerves, whose nuclei are situated in the midbrain and whose axons go out to supply five of the six eyeball muscles and the levator palpebrae superioris; and the trigeminal (V), the abducens (VI), and the facial (VII) nerves, all of which are found in the pons. The trigeminal nerve innervates the muscles of mastication, the abducens supplies the last remaining eyeball muscle, and the facial nerve, as its name implies, supplies all the muscles of facial expression. Finally, in the medulla are situated: the nucleus of the glossopharyngeal nerve (IX), which innervates a single muscle in the throat; the nucleus of the vagus nerve (X), which supplies muscles in the throat concerned with talking (the nucleus of IX and X is really a single, common nucleus called the *nucleus ambiguus*); the nucleus of the hypoglossal nerve (XII), which supplies all the muscles of the tongue; and the accessory nerve (XI), which is an exception in that it doesn't supply muscles in the head but two very important ones in the neck — the sternomastoid and the trapezius.

No mention has yet been made of the crossing-over of the corticobulbar tract because it isn't the

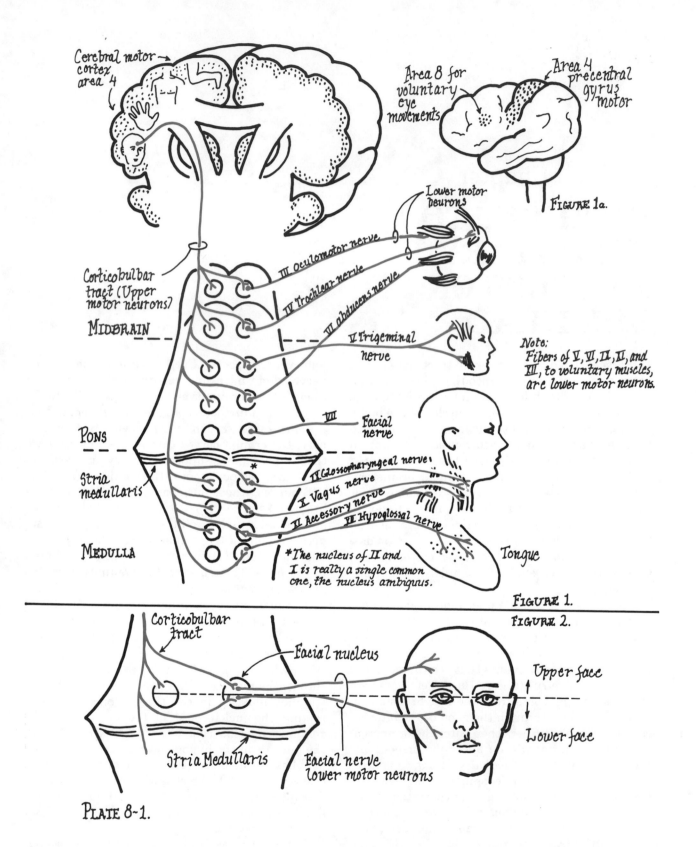

Cerebral motor cortex area 4

Area 8 for voluntary eye movements

Area 4 precentral gyrus motor

FIGURE 1a.

Lower motor neurons

Corticobulbar tract (Upper motor neurons)

MIDBRAIN

III Oculomotor nerve

IV Trochlear nerve

VI abducens nerve

V Trigeminal nerve

Note:
Fibers of V, VI, IV, III, and XII, to voluntary muscles, are lower motor neurons.

PONS

VII Facial nerve

Stria medullaris

IX Glossopharyngeal nerve

X Vagus nerve

XI Accessory nerve

XII Hypoglossal nerve

MEDULLA

*The nucleus of X and IX is really a single common one, the nucleus ambiguus.

Tongue

FIGURE 1.

FIGURE 2.

Corticobulbar tract

Facial nucleus

Upper face

Lower face

Stria Medullaris

Facial nerve lower motor neurons

PLATE 8-1.

same for all the cranial nerves just mentioned. The motor nuclei of all the cranial nerves mentioned, except VII and XII, receive innervation from both the right and left corticobulbar tracts, i.e., each corticobulbar tract supplies both the right and left cranial nuclei (Figure 1). This bilateral innervation is a kind of biological "insurance," e.g., if the right tract is damaged then the nuclei will still receive the upper motor neuron impulses from the intact left corticobulbar tract and there'll be no impairment of muscle function.

The nuclei of cranial nerve XII, the hypoglossal nerve, receive only contralateral innervation, i.e., the nucleus of the right side is supplied by axons from the left corticobulbar tract and vice versa. The clinical implication is fairly obvious: a lesion to the left corticobulbar tract would result in loss of nerve supply to the right nucleus and the muscles of the right side of the tongue would be paralyzed.

The facial nucleus, cranial nerve VII, combines features of both types of nuclei discussed so far. Its nucleus is divided into an upper part, which supplies the muscles of the upper half of the face, and a lower part, which supplies muscles in the lower half. The upper part of the nucleus receives bilateral innervation from the corticobulbar tract, while the lower part receives its supply from the contralateral tract (Figure 2).

CLINICAL ASPECTS

Upper Motor Neuron Lesion

As we have just seen, all the cranial motor nuclei (except the lower part of the facial and hypoglossal nerves) receive bilateral innervation. Therefore, if there is a lesion in one of the corticobulbar tracts, none of the nuclei or the muscles they supply would be affected. However an upper motor neuron lesion (also known as a supranuclear lesion) would affect XII and/or the lower part of VII. If corticobulbar fibers to the facial nucleus are damaged, there is paralysis of the lower part of the facial muscles on the side opposite the lesion (Figure 2). The paralysis is spastic, and reflexes are present. Since the upper part of the facial muscles receives bilateral innervation the patient can still move the brow on the paralyzed side of the face (Figure 2). If corticobulbar neurons to the hypoglossal nucleus are destroyed, the tongue muscles on the contralateral side will be paralyzed but they won't atrophy (Figure 1). When the patient is asked to protrude the tongue, the muscles on the unaffected side cause it to deviate to the side on which the muscles are paralyzed.

Lower Motor Neuron Lesions

Lower motor neuron lesions are discussed in Chapter 13, "Cranial Nerves."

Chapter 9

SUBCORTICAL MOTOR AREAS

In lower forms of animals, such as sharks and birds, which don't have a cerebral motor cortex, movement is initiated by a group of nuclei, the basal ganglia, together with other subcortical areas. Such movement is highly coordinated and often very quick, but it is instinctive and crude. In man there has been added to this old motor system a new, "higher" one — the cerebral motor cortex — which enables him to perform exceptionally skilled and purposeful movements, especially with his hands. This new system is called the pyramidal system, while the older, cruder one is the extrapyramidal system. For a while it was thought that the two were independent of each other, but now it's known that they are interconnected. Our knowledge of the old system is very incomplete, and a lot of what we think today may have to be modified by new discoveries tomorrow. With respect to terminology, there has been a tendency recently to use terms other than pyramidal and extrapyramidal, but this change in semantics hasn't been accompanied by any great increase in understanding. Also, many of the nuclei are grouped together and given special names, e.g., corpus striatum, lentiform nuclei. Since different authors don't always mean the same thing by the same term, the present author will name the nuclei and areas individually.

Deep in the cerebral hemisphere are three well-defined nuclei: the *caudate nucleus,* which lies medial to the anterior limb of the internal capsule, and the *globus pallidus* and *putamen,* which lie lateral to the genu (Figure 1). (These three plus the amygdala are the basal ganglia.) In the diencephalon is located the subthalamic nucleus of Luys, while in the midbrain are the red nucleus, the substantia nigra, and the reticular formation (Figure 2). All the above-mentioned structures make up the subcortical or primitive motor areas.

Various areas of the cerebral motor cortex, including areas, 4, 4s, and 6 send fibers to the caudate, putamen, and pallidus (Figure 3). The globus pallidus, which also receives fibers from the caudate and putamen, is the main discharge center and is therefore connected with the subthalamic nucleus, substantia nigra, reticular formation, and red nucleus (Figure 3). In addition, the subthalamic nucleus and substantia nigra are connected to the reticular formation and red nucleus, which discharge to the lower motor neurons at all levels of the cord via the reticulospinal and rubrospinal tracts (Figure 3). Thus, there is, as was so aptly described by the neuroanatomist Elliot, a "cascading effect" with respect to nuclei and their discharges. Finally, it should be mentioned that the globus pallidus is connected to the thalamus by two tracts, the *ansa lenticularis* and the *lenticular fasciculus.* As they enter the thalamus these two tracts merge to form the *thalamic fasciculus.* The thalamus in turn is connected back to the caudate and areas 4, 4s, and 6, thus establishing a "feedback" mechanism. If our knowledge of the interconnections between different subcortical nuclei plus their relationship to areas 4, 4s, and 6 is poor, then our understanding of how they operate and regulate motor activity is almost nil.

CLINICAL ASPECTS

Lesions in the primitive subcortical nuclei produce several diseases characterized by disturbances of muscle tone and various abnormal involuntary movements (dyskinesia). The most common and best known disease is *Parkinsonism.* Clinically, one sees a great increase in muscle tonus, leading to rigidity and slowness of movement. Combined with this is tremor, seen especially in the arms and hands, where it manifests itself in a characteristic pill-rolling motion. This tremor is most evident when the patient isn't doing anything with his hands — a resting tremor — but often disappears during purposeful movements. During walking, the head and shoulders are stooped, the gait is short and shuffling, and there is a loss of automatic movements, such as swinging of the arms. The face loses all signs of expression and becomes mask-like. The cause of the

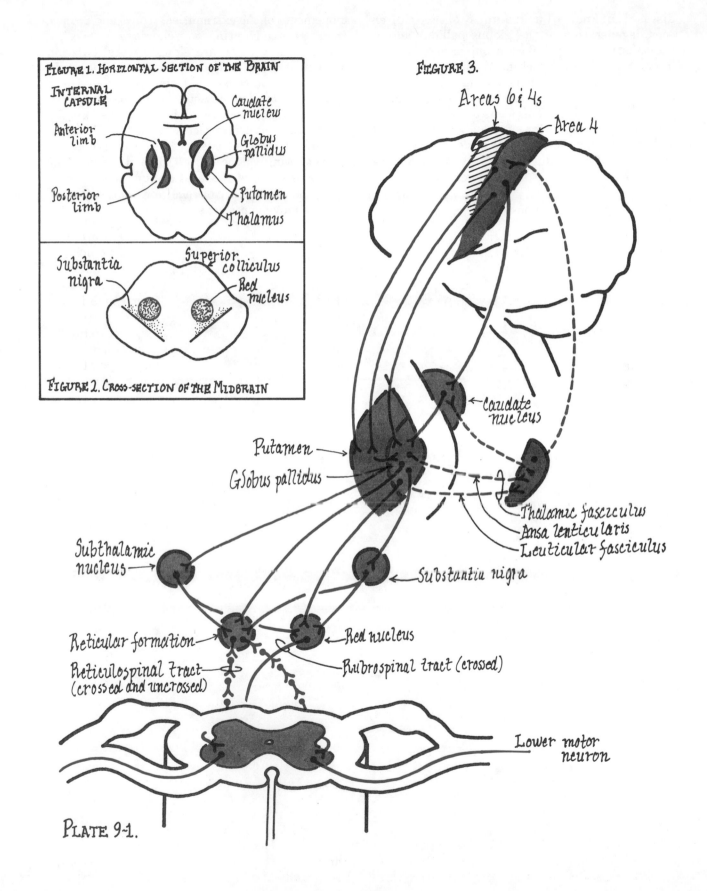

FIGURE 1. HORIZONTAL SECTION OF THE BRAIN

INTERNAL CAPSULE

Anterior limb

Posterior limb

Caudate nucleus

Globus pallidus

Putamen

Thalamus

Substantia nigra

Superior colliculus

Red nucleus

FIGURE 2. CROSS-SECTION OF THE MIDBRAIN

FIGURE 3.

Areas 6 & 4s

Area 4

Caudate nucleus

Putamen

Globus pallidus

Thalamic fasciculus

Ansa lenticularis

Lenticular fasciculus

Subthalamic nucleus

Substantia nigra

Reticular formation

Reticulospinal tract (crossed and uncrossed)

Red nucleus

Rubrospinal tract (crossed)

Lower motor neuron

PLATE 9-1.

disease is unknown, but at autopsy one most often sees degeneration of the globus pallidus and/or the substantia nigra. Parkinsonism may be seen in other conditions, such as Wilson's disease, in which there is abnormal copper metabolism that results in copper deposition in the globus pallidus, putamen, and liver. This causes their degeneration and the production of the above-mentioned symptoms. In mental patients high doses of chlorpromazine often produce signs of Parkinsonism as a temporary and unpleasant side effect.

Huntington's chorea is a condition characterized by rapid, jerky, non-rhythmic, involuntary movements of the extremities, trunk, and/or face. In contrast to Huntington's chorea, *athetosis* is a disease where there are slow, bizzare, twisting movements, especially in the arms and fingers. In these two conditions the lesion isn't found in a specific subcortical nucleus, i.e., it may be in the caudate or putamen or globus pallidus. Lastly, there is *hemiballism,* which is caused by a lesion in the subthalamic nucleus. In this disease there is a violent swinging motion of the arm or leg. The causes of all three diseases are unknown. Tragically, there is no cure or relief for these sufferers, and the movements cease only in sleep.

Chapter 10

THE VESTIBULAR SYSTEM

It happens to all of us — suddenly, for one reason or another, one loses one's balance, starts to fall, and immediately a reflex reaction known as a "righting mechanism" comes into play in an attempt to regain equilibrium. This sense of loss of equilibrium and the reflex mechanisms to regain and maintain it are the function of the vestibular division of the eighth cranial nerve, the acousto-vestibular nerve. The vestibular system is considered part of the extrapyramidal network because it doesn't involve the cerebral motor cortex and its actions are reflexive.

The receptor organ is located in the inner ear and consists of two fluid-filled sacs, the *utricle* and the *sacculus,* and three fluid-filled semicircular canals lying perpendicular to each other, which represent the three spatial planes (Figure 1). The fluid is *endolymph,* and suspended in it are specialized receptor cells — the *hair cells* — which are sensitive to fluid currents. When there is a shift or change of position of the head, the endolymph is set in motion; it stimulates the receptors, which transmit this information to the brain, which in turn sets off the appropriate reflex responses.

From the inner ear, 1° neurons pass to the brain, with their cell bodies aggregated in the vestibular ganglion. Axons leave this ganglion and enter the brainstem, where they terminate in four vestibular nuclei situated in the area acoustica of the floor of the fourth ventricle (Figure 1). These nuclei have five major connections, which are discussed below one by one.

VESTIBULOCEREBELLAR CONNECTIONS

The cerebellum is the coordination center for motor activity and equilibrium. Therefore, from the superior and lateral vestibular nuclei, 2° neurons pass up into the cerebellum via its inferior peduncle and terminate in the flocculonodular lobe (Figure 1). In addition, there are a few 1° axons that don't end in the vestibular nuclei, but pass directly to the floccular nodulus (Figure 1). This then discharges back to the vestibular nuclei of *both sides* via the fastigial nucleus and the inferior peduncle — thus, a cerebellar-vestibular feedback mechanism is established (Figure 1).

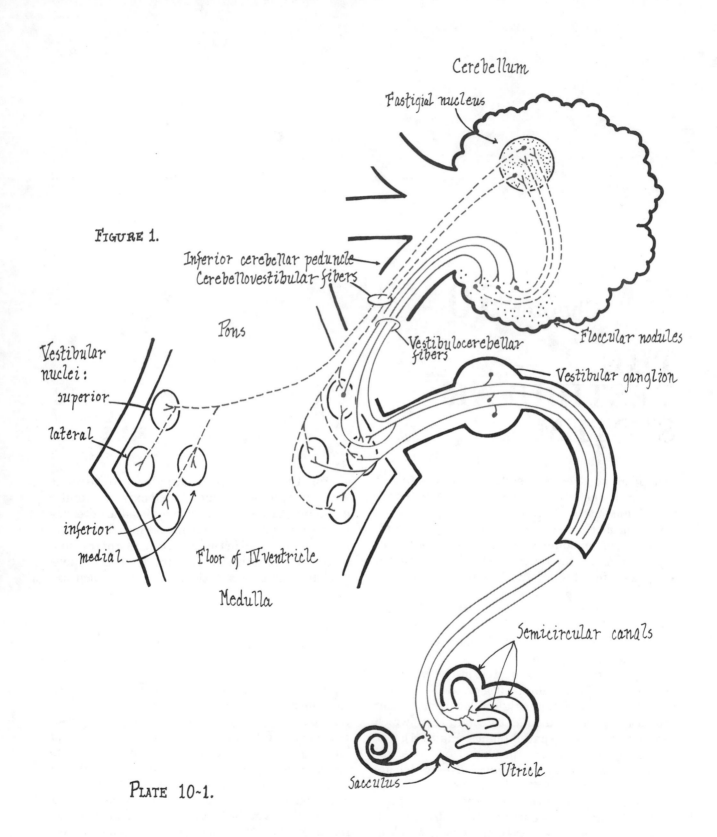

Cerebellum

Fastigial nucleus

FIGURE 1.

Inferior cerebellar peduncle
Cerebellovestibular fibers

Pons

Vestibulocerebellar fibers

Floccular nodules

Vestibular ganglion

Vestibular nuclei:

superior

lateral

inferior

medial

Floor of IV ventricle

Medulla

Semicircular canals

Sacculus

Utricle

PLATE 10-1.

VESTIBULOSPINAL TRACTS

From the lateral vestibular nucleus, secondary neurons descend in the ipsilateral ventral white volumn and end by synapsing on lower motor neurons. These 2° neurons, which discharge reflexively to maintain equilibrium, form the lateral vestibulospinal tract (Figure 2). (Lateral here refers not to the fact that it originates in the lateral nucleus, but to the fact that it lies lateral to the medial vestibulospinal tract, which is discussed next.)

From the medial, superior, and inferior vestibular nuclei, 2° crossed and uncrossed neurons descend in the ventral white columns and terminate on lower motor neurons. These secondary neurons, which form the medial vestibulospinal tracts, also discharge reflexively to maintain body equilibrium (Figure 2).

VESTIBULO-OCULAR CONNECTIONS

Besides helping to maintain body equilibrium, the vestibular system also has the function of regulating eyeball movements in certain cases. For example, if one looks straight ahead and fixes one's eyes on an object and then turns one's head to the side, the appropriate eyeball muscles must contract in order for the eyes to remain "locked in" on the object. The regulation or control of this contraction is a function of the vestibular system. It works as follows: When one turns one's head, the endolymph in the semicircular canals, sacculus, and utricle is set in motion and stimulates the hair cells. This stimulus passes via the nerve and vestibular ganglion to the vestibular nuclei. We just mentioned that, from the medial, superior, and inferior nuclei, crossed and uncrossed neurons descend as the medial vestibulospinal tract. Just before descending, these neurons branch and give off axons that ascend in the pons and midbrain, where they synapse in the sixth (abducens), fourth (trochlear), and third (oculomotor) nuclei, which are all concerned with eyeball muscle movement. These ascending axons regulate the amount of eyeball muscle contraction, and form the medial longitudinal fasciculus (the MLF) (Figure 2). (Some neuroanatomy books refer to the lateral vestibulospinal tract as the vestibulospinal tract, while the vestibulospinal tract is called the medial longitudinal fasciculus, or MLF.)

VESTIBULOCORTICAL CONNECTIONS

We can all sense a loss of equilibrium, or dizziness, if we are spun around quickly. This sensation implies vestibular connections to the thalamus, cerebral cortex, and consciousness. However, until now no such connections have been demonstrated morphologically. Some evidence has been obtained from electrophysiological studies, but the problem remains unsolved.

ACCESSORY PATHWAY

We mentioned above that the fastigial nucleus of the cerebellum is part of the feedback mechanism to the vestibular nuclei, which then discharge to the lower motor neurons via the lateral and medial vestibulospinal tracts. There is, in addition, another pathway to maintain equilibrium. The fastigial nucleus is connected to the descending reticular areas and nuclei of the brainstem, which then discharge to the lower motor neurons via the multisynaptic reticulospinal tract (see Figure 3 in the next chapter, "The Cerebellum," and also Chapter 18, on the reticular systems).

CLINICAL ASPECTS

Lesions of the vestibular system produce disturbances in equilibrium and walking straight, and, since this system is connected with eyeball movements, abnormal to-and-fro movements of the eyes, known as *nystagmus*. In nystagmus the eyes are constantly moving: first they move to one side as far as they can go, and then they snap back very quickly, then again they move slowly, etc. There is thus a slow movement to one side and a quick one to the other; the nystagmus is called left or right nystagmus according to the direction of the quick movement. Most nystagmi are horizontal in direction, but one can also have vertical nystagmus. Nystagmus is also very often seen in albinos.

Normal nystagmus can be seen in persons riding on trains. While they are looking out the window, their eyes will automatically focus on an object, follow it slowly until it's out of sight, and then snap back quickly and focus on another object. This slow-fast pattern of movement is repeated. Nystagmus is a complex phenomenon, and an excellent discussion of it, as well as of the vestibular system, can be found in Chapter 13 of *A Functional Approach to Neuroanatomy,* by House and Pansky (McGraw-Hill, 1960).

Another common symptom of vestibular injury is dizziness, although other conditions can also produce it. *Ménière's disease* is a disease of unknown etiology in which the patient suffers attacks of dizziness, ringing in the ears, and deafness.

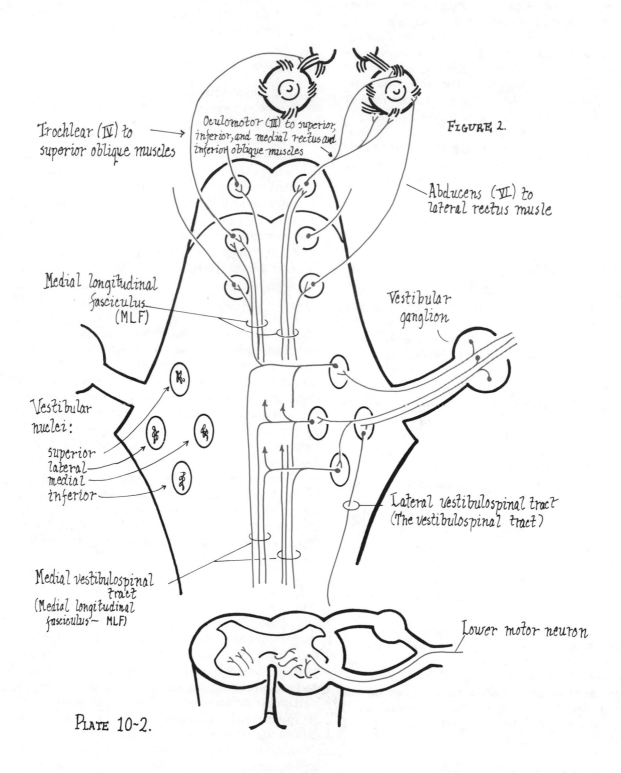

Trochlear (IV) to superior oblique muscles

Oculomotor (III) to superior, inferior, and medial rectus and inferior oblique muscles

FIGURE 2.

Abducens (VI) to lateral rectus musle

Medial longitudinal fasciculus (MLF)

Vestibular ganglion

Vestibular nuclei:
   superior
   lateral
   medial
   inferior

Lateral vestibulospinal tract (The vestibulospinal tract)

Medial vestibulospinal tract (Medial longitudinal fasciculus~ MLF)

Lower motor neuron

PLATE 10~2.

Chapter 11

THE CEREBELLUM AND ITS PATHWAYS

The cerebellum is the control center for the coordination of voluntary muscle activity, equilibrium, and muscle tonus. It does not initiate movement; therefore, a person who has cerebellar injury isn't paralyzed. Rather, his or her movements are slow, clumsy, tremulous, and uncoordinated. The muscles may be hypertonic or hypotonic and the person is unable to walk steadily, but tends to sway, stagger, and fall. In order to carry out its three important functions, the cerebellum needs to receive a steady stream of information concerning:

1. the position and state of the muscles and joints, and the amount of tonus present
2. the equilibrium state of the body
3. what "orders" are being sent to the muscles from the cerebral motor cortex.

Receiving these three information "inputs," the cerebellum is then able to integrate them and, by means of "feedback" pathways, regulate and control — automatically and at an unconscious level — motor activity, equilibrium, and muscle tonus. The discussion in this chapter considers each of the information "inputs" separately and then presents the "feedback" pathways.

THE SPINOCEREBELLAR PATHWAYS

Information concerning the condition of the muscles, the amount of tonus, and the position of the body is supplied by unconscious proprioceptive fibers, whose receptors are found in joints, tendons, and muscles. The cell bodies of these neurons are situated in the dorsal root ganglion and the axons pass into the cord, from which they can reach the cerebellum by either one of two tracts. Most of those from the lower part of the body enter the dorsal horn, where they synapse with 2° neurons (Figure 1). Some of these secondary neurons ascend on the same side, in the ventral spinocerebellar tract of the lateral columns, and enter the cerebellum through its superior peduncle. The remaining secondary axons cross over to the contralateral side, enter the ventral spinocerebellar tract there and ascend to the cerebellum. However, before passing into the superior cerebellar peduncle they cross back to the side from which they started (Figure 1).

Proprioceptive fibers from the upper part of the body use the dorsal spinocerebellar tract. Here primary neurons synapse with secondary ones in Clarke's nucleus (Figure 1), which is found only in the upper part of the spinal cord. Secondary axons pass into the lateral columns on the same side to form the dorsal spinocerebellar tract, which enters the cerebellum through the inferior cerebellar peduncle. The important thing to remember is that all spinocerebellar fibers enter the cerebellum on the same side that they entered the cord.

The dorsal and ventral spinocerebellar tracts are the main bundles supplying proprioceptive impulses to the cerebellum. There are, however, a number of others, such as the trigeminocerebellar tract, from the muscles of mastication and the mandibular joint, and the olivocerebellar tract, as well as the reticulocerebellar and arcuocerebellar tracts.

33

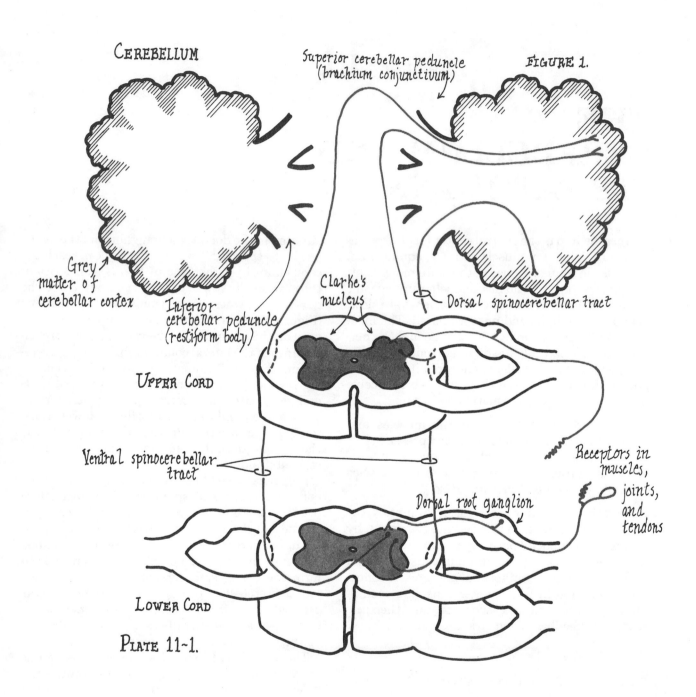

CEREBELLUM
Superior cerebellar peduncle
(brachium conjunctivum)
FIGURE 1.

Grey matter of cerebellar cortex

Inferior cerebellar peduncle (restiform body)

Clarke's nucleus

Dorsal spinocerebellar tract

UPPER CORD

Ventral spinocerebellar tract

Dorsal root ganglion

Receptors in muscles, joints, and tendons

LOWER CORD

PLATE 11~1.

VESTIBULOCEREBELLAR TRACT

From the superior and lateral vestibular nuclei arise the fibers that supply information concerning the equilibrium state of the body. They enter through the ipsilateral (homolateral) inferior peduncle and pass to the cerebellar cortex, especially of the flocculus (Figure 2). Phylogenetically, the flocculus is the oldest part of the cerebellum and a center for equilibrium.

CORTICOPONTOCEREBELLAR TRACTS

When the cerebral motor cortex discharges to the lower motor neurons, the cerebellum must receive information about the nature of the discharge, i.e., to what muscles it is going, how strong it is, etc., and it gets this information through the corticopontocerebellar tracts. The fibers originate in the cerebral cortex, descend through the internal capsule, and, at the level of the pons, synapse with 2° neurons in the pontine nuclei (Figure 2). The secondary axons now cross over the the other side and enter the cerebellum through its middle peduncle.

"FEEDBACK PATHWAYS"

The cerebellum, having received information concerning muscle states, tonus, and equilibrium, as well as the nature of the motor discharge to the muscles, integrates all this "input" (how, we don't know) and exerts its control via the following pathways:

From the cerebellar cortex, short neurons pass to several cerebellar nuclei, the emboliform, fastigial, globus, and dentate nuclei. The last-named nucleus is the most important; it sends out fibers through the superior peduncle that decussate and then enter the red nucleus of the midbrain (Figure 3). Not surprisingly, they are called the *dentorubro fibers,* or the dentatorubrothalamic tract, since some of them bypass the red nucleus and go up to the thalamus. The red nucleus can discharge up to the thalamus, which relays the information up to the cerebral motor cortex; thus the "feedback" circuit is completed (Figure 3). The red nu-

cleus can also discharge down to the lower motor neuron by means of the rubrospinal tract (Figure 3), and thus can influence the corticospinal impulses at the spinal level.

The cerebellum also discharges back, directly or through the fastigial nucleus, to the vestibular nuclei. These in turn relay the stimuli to the lower motor neurons by means of the vestibulospinal tract (Figure 3).

Finally, the cerebellum can influence the lower motor neurons by discharging to the reticular area and nuclei of the pons, and midbrain, and medulla, which relay the discharge by the lateral and medial reticulospinal tract (Figure 3).

CLINICAL ASPECTS

Lesions of the cerebellum or its afferent and efferent tracts produce several characteristic signs, usually on the same side of the body as the injury:

1. *Asynergia* is the loss of coordination in performing motor acts. One sees decomposition of movement, i.e., it is done in jerky stages instead of smoothly.
2. *Dysmetria* is the inability to judge distance and to stop movement at a chosen spot. Thus, in reaching for an object, a patient's hand will over- or under-reach it; or, when he is asked to touch the tip of his nose, his finger will hit his cheek — a pass-pointing phenomena.
3. *Adiadochokinesia* is the inability to perform rapidly alternating movements, such as pronation and supination of the hands.
4. *Intention tremor* occurs during a movement and not at rest. In Parkinson's disease one sees just the opposite — a resting tremor.
5. *Ataxia* means abnormal gait; the person staggers and reels. To compensate, he walks with the feet spread apart.
6. *Falling* — The patient has a tendency to fall, especially to the injured side.
7. *Hypotonia* — The muscles are floppy and weak, but may be hypertonic in some cases.
8. *Dysphonia* is a slurred, explosive speech.
9. *Nystagmus* may be present.

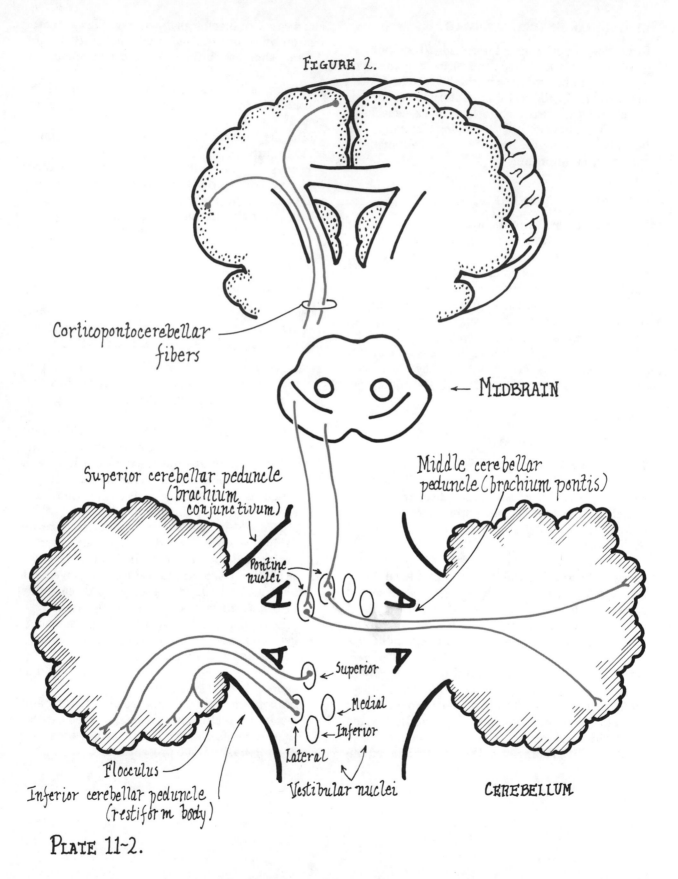

FIGURE 2.

Corticopontocerebellar fibers

← MIDBRAIN

Superior cerebellar peduncle (brachium conjunctivum)

Middle cerebellar peduncle (brachium pontis)

Pontine nuclei

Superior

Medial

Inferior

Lateral

Vestibular nuclei

Flocculus

Inferior cerebellar peduncle (restiform body)

CEREBELLUM

PLATE 11-2.

FIGURE 3.

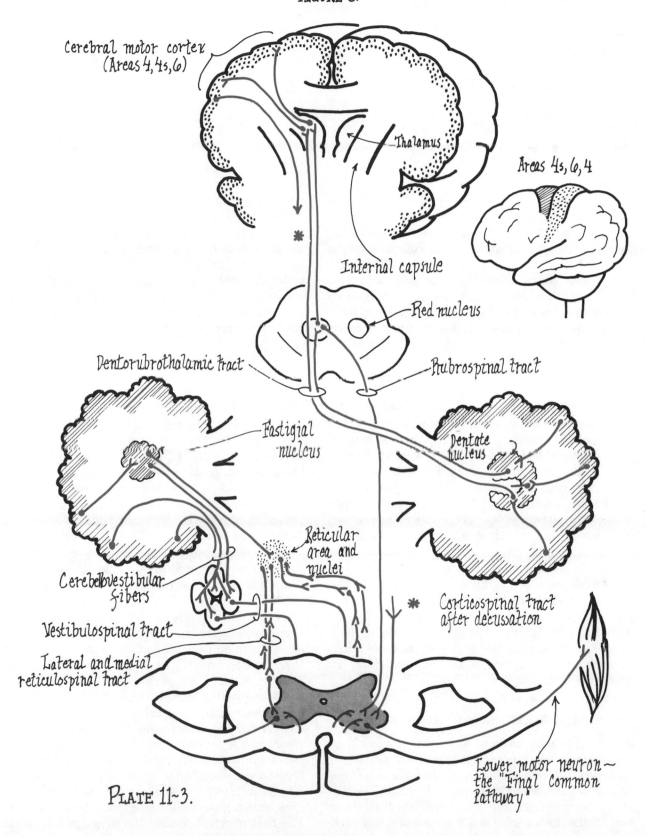

Cerebral motor cortex
(Areas 4, 4s, (6))

Thalamus

Areas 4s, 6, 4

Internal capsule

Red nucleus

Dentorubrothalamic tract

Rubrospinal tract

Fastigial
nucleus

Dentate
nucleus

Reticular
area and
nuclei

Cerebellovestibular
fibers

Corticospinal tract
after decussation

Vestibulospinal tract

Lateral and medial
reticulospinal tract

Lower motor neuron~
the "Final Common
Pathway"

PLATE 11~3.

Chapter 12

THE AUTONOMIC NERVOUS SYSTEM

The autonomic nervous system (ANS) stimulates and controls structures not under conscious control. If, for example, you are suddenly told that you're getting a surprise exam, your heart rate will probably increase, your mouth will go dry, you'll get "butterflies" in your stomach, and you'll start sweating — all automatic reactions to a stress situation. The autonomic nervous system stimulates three types of tissues: cardiac muscle, most glands, and all smooth muscle (found in many organs and structures). It is divided into two parts, the *sympathetic* nervous system and the *parasympathetic* nervous system, both of which supply (with two or three exceptions) the same organs and structures. However, they are antagonistic to each other, e.g., sympathetic stimulation of the heart results in an increased pulse rate, while parasympathetic stimulation slows it down. Or, with respect to pupil size, sympathetic discharge results in dilation, while parasympathetic stimulation produces constriction. The two systems are constantly discharging to the structures they supply, but there is a balance between them (Figure 1a). This balance can be changed in either of two ways. First, by increasing the amount of stimulus in one part of the autonomic nervous system (Figure 1b) or by decreasing the amount of discharge in the other (Figure 1c). This very important principle forms the basis of much of neuropharmacology; it is discussed later in greater detail.

THE SYMPATHETIC NERVOUS SYSTEM

The sympathetic nervous system is the one that dominates when a person is in a stress situation, be it physical or psychological. In both instances one feels threatened, and the body automatically reacts by preparing for "fight or flight." In these conditions the muscles will work harder, will need more oxygen, and will use more energy. Therefore, the bronchioles open up for quicker and greater passage of air; the heart beats stronger and faster; the arteries to the heart and voluntary muscles dilate, thereby bringing more blood to them; the arteries to the skin and peripheral areas of the body constrict, thereby shunting more blood to the active muscles (and as a result the skin feels cold); the liver secretes glycogen for quick supply of energy; peristalsis slows down, since the body has no energy or time for digestion; the pupils dilate to get a better view of the surroundings; the hair "stands on end"; and one sweats. The last two are interesting evolutionary carryovers of more primitive defense reactions. The hairs of a cat that's threatened by a dog stand up so that if the dog attempts to bite the body it'll get a mouthful of hairs instead. As for sweating, did you ever try to grab and hold a person who is wet and slippery?

The sympathetic nervous system is based on a two-neuron pathway. The cell bodies of the first neurons are located in the lateral gray horn of the spinal cord, which is situated only between the first thoracic segment and the third lumbar T_1-L_3 (Figure 2) (and the system is also called the thoracolumbar outflow). The axons leave the cord via the ventral roots and enter the sympathetic trunk. The sympathetic trunk is a series of ganglia and axon fibers on each side of the vertebral column that extends from the neck to the sacrum. It is also referred to as the paravertebral chain ganglia or the sympathetic chain. The question is, how do the primary axons that exit at thoracic 1 (T_1) reach the glands and smooth-muscled structures up in the head? After entering the sympathetic trunk the axons ascend in it until they reach the superior cervical ganglion in the upper region of the neck (Figure 2). Here they synapse with secondary neurons, which go out and innervate the glands, etc. The first neuron is called the preganglionic fiber

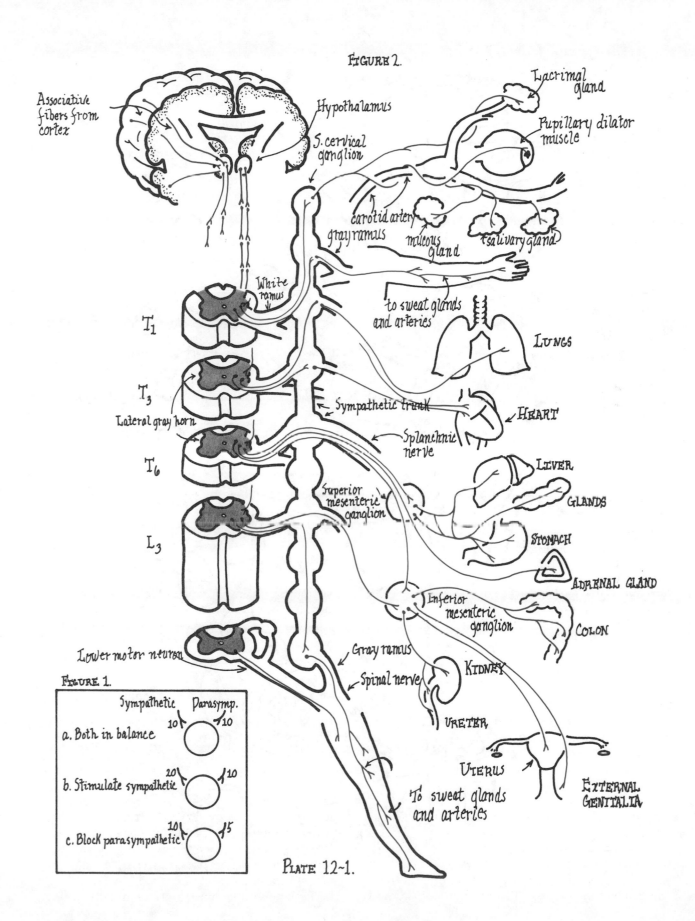

FIGURE 2.

Associative fibers from cortex

Hypothalamus

Lacrimal gland

Pupillary dilator muscle

S. cervical ganglion

carotid artery
gray ramus

mucous gland

salivary gland

White ramus

T_1

to sweat glands and arteries

LUNGS

T_3

Sympathetic trunk

HEART

Lateral gray horn

Splanchnic nerve

T_6

LIVER

Superior mesenteric ganglion

GLANDS

STOMACH

L_3

ADRENAL GLAND

Inferior mesenteric ganglion

COLON

Lower motor neuron

Gray ramus

KIDNEY

Spinal nerve

FIGURE 1.

URETER

	Sympathetic	Parasymp.
a. Both in balance	10	10
b. Stimulate sympathetic	20	10
c. Block parasympathetic	10	5

UTERUS

To sweat glands and arteries

EXTERNAL GENITALIA

PLATE 12~1.

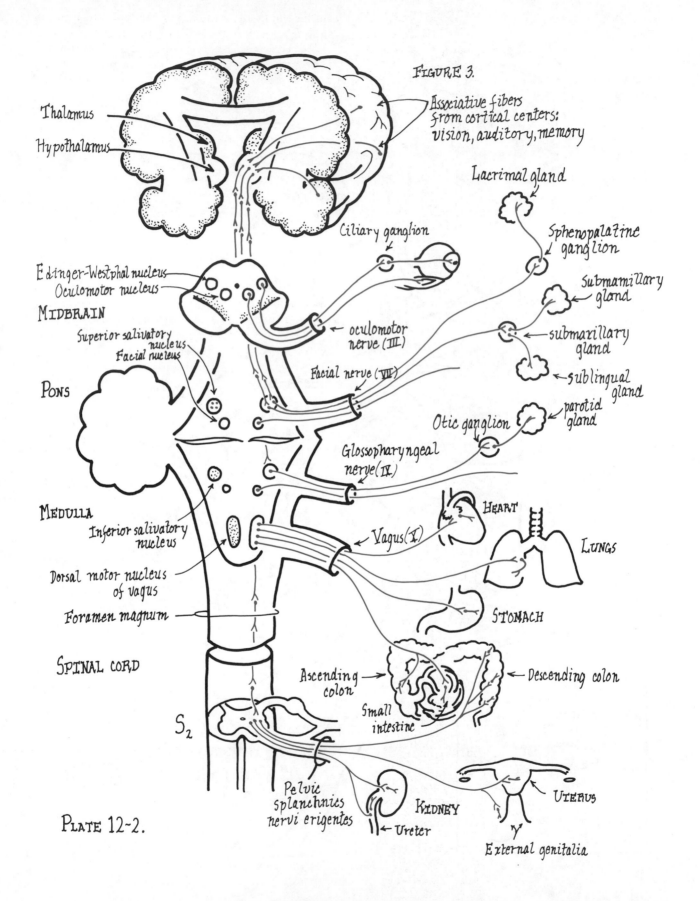

FIGURE 3.

Thalamus

Hypothalamus

Associative fibers from cortical centers: vision, auditory, memory

Lacrimal gland

Ciliary ganglion

Sphenopalatine ganglion

Edinger-Westphal nucleus
Oculomotor nucleus

MIDBRAIN

Submamillary gland

oculomotor nerve (III)

submaxillary gland

Superior salivatory nucleus
Facial nucleus

Facial nerve (VII)

sublingual gland

PONS

parotid gland

Otic ganglion

Glossopharyngeal nerve (IX)

MEDULLA

Inferior salivatory nucleus

HEART

Vagus (X)

LUNGS

Dorsal motor nucleus of vagus

STOMACH

Foramen magnum

SPINAL CORD

Ascending colon

Descending colon

Small intestine

S₂

Pelvic splanchnics nervi erigentes

KIDNEY

UTERUS

Ureter

External genitalia

PLATE 12-2.

and its axon is myelinated, while the second is the postganglionic fiber and its axon is unmyelinated. This postganglionic axon reaches its "destination" by leaving the superior cervical ganglion and wrapping itself around the arteries that reach the innervated structures. Or, one might say, it "hitches a ride" on the arteries until it comes to the glands and smooth-muscled structures and then it peels off to innervate them (Figure 2).

Cell bodies of sympathetics destined to supply the heart and lungs are situated in the lateral gray horn of segments T_1–T_5. The axons leave the cord and enter the chain ganglia, where they synapse with postganglionic neurons (Figure 2). The axons of the latter leave the chain ganglia and form specific nerves that reach the heart and lungs (Figure 2).

Those sympathetics that supply the abdominal viscera are found in the lateral horn of T_6–T_{12}. Their axons enter the chain ganglia, but they don't synapse there. Rather, they pass through it and leave to form distinct nerves, the splanchnics, which terminate in the superior and inferior mesenteric ganglions of the abdomen (Figure 2). The postganglionic axons leave and form a net-like plexus that spreads out to reach the various organs. Some of the preganglionic axons pass to the adrenal gland, the medullary cells of which *are* the postganglionic neurons that are specialized to secrete the hormone adrenaline (Figure 2).

Most of the preganglionics to the kidneys and pelvic organs are located in the lateral horn of spinal segments L_1–L_3 (Figure 2). Their axons enter the sympathetic chain, pass through it without synapsing, and descend to end in the inferior mesenteric ganglion. From here the postganglionics fan out to supply the urinary and genital organs (Figure 2).

Accessory Detail

The preganglionic axons are myelinated and are therefore white. They leave the cord, and to get to the sympathetic chain they peel off from the spinal nerve and form the white ramus communicantes, which links up the two (Figure 2). The postganglionic axons are unmyelinated and therefore appear gray. Many rejoin the spinal nerves through the gray ramus communicantes and pass out to supply the sweat glands and peripheral arteries of the upper extremity, the trunk, and the lower limbs (Figure 2).

The chemical transmitter between the postganglionic sympathetic axons and the structures they innervate is not acetylcholine, but adrenaline. If a patient is given a shot of adrenaline, the reaction is the same as if the sympathetic nervous system had discharged. Consequently, this system is also called the *adrenergic nervous system*. There are drugs that block the parasympathetic system from discharging, which results in an imbalance between the two parts of the autonomic nervous system, and what one sees is similar in many ways to what happens when the sympathetics discharge (Figure 1c). Among the best-known parasympathetic blocking agents is *atropine* (Bella donna), which causes marked pupillary dilation and is therefore used by ophthalmologists when they want to take a good look at the eye.

THE PARASYMPATHETIC NERVOUS SYSTEM

This system is also based on a two-neuron pathway, consisting of preganglionic and postganglionic neurons. However, there are great physiological, anatomical, and pharmacological differences between the two systems. Whereas the sympathetic nervous system is dominant in stress situations, the parasympathetic is most active when a person is relaxed and resting; the heart beat slows down, peristalsis and other digestive functions are active, etc.

As for the anatomy, the preganglionic cell bodies are located in the brainstem and in the gray matter of the cord in the sacral region. Therefore another name for this system is the cranial-sacral outflow. In the brainstem the cell bodies are aggregated in several specific nuclei and the axons join the third, seventh, ninth, and tenth cranial nerves. Being components of these nerves, they exit with them, pass out to the different regions, and, very near their destinations, enter specific-named ganglia. Here the preganglionic axons synapse with short postganglionic fibers that innervate glands, the heart, and structures having smooth muscle. In many cases the ganglia are situated near, on, or within the structures innervated and the postganglionic fibers are microscopic.

At the level of the superior colliculus of the midbrain, preganglionic cell bodies are located in the *Edinger-Westphal nucleus* (Figure 3). The axons join the lower motor fibers of the oculomotor nerve (cranial nerve III) and together they leave the midbrain and course out to the eyeball (Figure 3). Near it, the preganglionic axons peel off and enter the ciliary ganglion, where they synapse with postganglionic neurons. These send out short axons to the pupillary constrictor muscle.

The preganglionic cell bodies associated with the seventh, or facial, nerve are situated in the superior salivatory nucleus and their axons pass out to the sphenopalatine and submaxillary ganglia (Figure 3). From here the postganglionic axons course out to the lacrimal gland, as well as to the sublingual and submaxillary glands.

As for the ninth cranial nerve, the glossopharyngeal, its preganglionic cell bodies are in the inferior salivatory nucleus and the axons go out to the otic ganglion, which sends out postganglionic fibers to the parotid gland (Figure 3).

The vagus nerve (cranial nerve X) is the most important cranial nerve because most of its fibers are parasympathetic neurons that innervate the heart, lungs, and all the abdominal viscera up to the left colic flexure. The preganglionic cell bodies are aggregated in the dorsal motor nucleus of the vagus and the axons pass out and terminate in ganglia situated in the walls of the above-mentioned organs (Figure 3). From these mural ganglia, microscopic postganglionic neurons innervate the structures.

The descending colon and the genital and urinary systems are supplied by the sacral outflow. Here the preganglionic cell bodies are situated in the lateral area of the gray matter of spinal segments sacral 2–4. The axons leave through the ventral roots and soon separate from the spinal nerve to form the pelvic splanchnic nerves or nervi erigentes, which reach the mural ganglia of the descending colon, kidney, ureter, and genital organs (Figure 3).

Accessory Detail

The chemical transmitter between the postganglionic parasympathetic axons and the structures they innervate is acetylcholine. Thus, if one gives a patient such a drug, the reaction resembles parasympathetic discharge.

The hypothalamus is the control and integrative center for the autonomic nervous system, and its actions are automatic and not regularly subject to conscious control. (The hypothalamus is part of the diencephalon and lies below the thalamus on either side of the third ventricle (Figure 3).) It receives fiber bundles mainly from higher cortical centers, such as vision, auditory, personality, etc., and then discharges the appropriate impulses down the cord to the sympathetic or parasympathetic preganglionic neurons. It does this by means of the dorsal longitudinal fasciculus, the mamillotegmental tract, and the multisynaptic reticulospinal tract (see Chapters 17 and 18 on the reticular formation and the hypothalamus).

Chapter **13**

CRANIAL NERVES

The 12 pairs of cranial nerves, which we have already discussed in passing in previous chapters, are considered in detail here. These nerves can be grouped in several ways, the first way being according to their central location (see figures in this chapter and also the Atlas). Cranial nerves I and II, the olfactory and optic nerves, are connected to the telencephalon; nerves III and IV, the oculomotor and trochlear nerves, are connected with the midbrain; the trigeminal (V), the abducens (VI), and the facial (VII) nerves are located in the pons; while the remaining nerves (VIII, IX, X, XI, and XII), are associated with the medulla. It's important to know this location plan: if a patient exhibits signs of a specific cranial nerve injury, then the site of the lesion can be pinpointed.

Another way to group cranial nerves is according to their functional neuronal components. Some have only sensory neurons; they are (Figure 1a):

I, the *olfactory* nerve, concerned with smell (see Chapter 16)
II, the *optic* nerve, which deals with vision (see Chapter 15)
VIII, the *acoustovestibular* nerve, concerned with hearing and equilibrium (see Chapters 10 and 14).

Other cranial nerves are composed only of motor neurons to voluntary muscles; they are (Figure 1b):

IV, the *trochlear* nerve, which innervates the superior oblique muscle of the eyeball. If the nerve or its nucleus is damaged, the muscle will be paralyzed and there'll be difficulty in turning the affected eye downward and laterally.

VI, the *abducens* nerve, which innervates the lateral rectus muscle of the eyeball. If this nerve or its nucleus is injured the muscle becomes paralyzed and the patient can't turn the eye laterally. In time, the unopposed medial rectus causes the eye to be pulled medially, thus producing a medial strabismus (squint).

XI, the *accessory* nerve, which innervates two important muscles outside the head: the trapezius and the sternocleidomastoid muscles. These two neck muscles are also supplied by spinal nerves; thus, if the accessory nerve or its nucleus is damaged, the muscles will still function partially. However, the patient will have difficulty shrugging the shoulder on the affected side and turning the head to the opposite side.

XII, the *hypoglossal* nerve, which supplies all the muscles of the tongue. Again, if this nerve or its nucleus is damaged then the muscles on the affected side become paralyzed, and the tongue, when it is protruded, will deviate to the paralyzed side. The reason for this is that tongue muscles are so arranged that, if one side is paralyzed, then, upon protrusion, the muscles on the unparalyzed side push the tongue over to the paralyzed side.

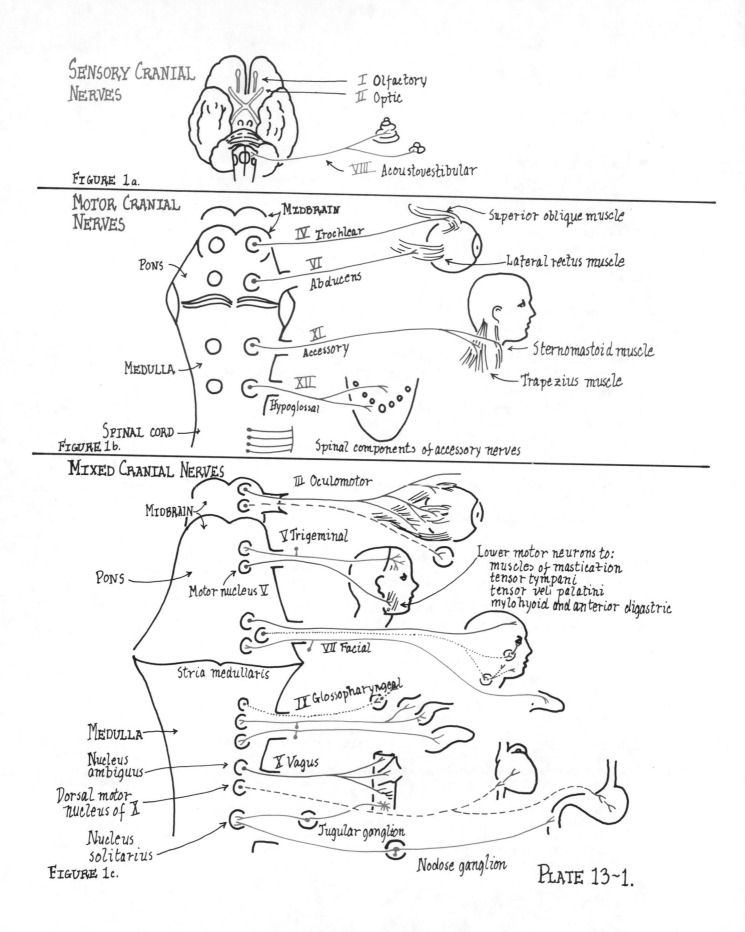

SENSORY CRANIAL NERVES

I Olfactory
II Optic

VIII Acoustovestibular

FIGURE 1a.

MOTOR CRANIAL NERVES

MIDBRAIN

IV Trochlear
Superior oblique muscle

PONS

VI Abducens
Lateral rectus muscle

MEDULLA

XI Accessory
Sternomastoid muscle
Trapezius muscle

XII Hypoglossal

SPINAL CORD

Spinal components of accessory nerves

FIGURE 1b.

MIXED CRANIAL NERVES

III Oculomotor

MIDBRAIN

V Trigeminal

PONS

Motor nucleus V

Lower motor neurons to:
muscles of mastication
tensor tympani
tensor veli palatini
mylohyoid and anterior digastric

VII Facial

Stria medullaris

IX Glossopharyngeal

MEDULLA

Nucleus ambiguus

X Vagus

Dorsal motor nucleus of X

Nucleus solitarius

Jugular ganglion

Nodose ganglion

FIGURE 1c.

PLATE 13~1.

Note: a very old mnemonic device for use in naming the 12 cranial nerves is:
"*On Old Olympus' Towering Top, A Finn And German Viewed A House*"

olfactory optic oculomotor trochlear trigeminal abducens facial acoustic glossopharyngeal vagus accessory hypoglossal

The remaining cranial nerves (III, V, VII, IX, and X) have mixed functional neuronal components (Figure 1c). Each of these mixed cranial nerves is discussed below in detail.

THE OCULOMOTOR NERVE (III)

The motor nucleus of the oculomotor nerve is located in the midbrain below the aqueduct of Sylvius at the level of the superior colliculus (Figure 2 and Atlas, Figure 10). From it emerge voluntary motor fibers (lower motor neurons), which leave the brainstem at the interpeduncular fossa and pass out to the orbit. Here they supply the following four eyeball muscles: the superior rectus, inferior rectus, and medial rectus muscles, and the inferior oblique muscle. In addition, they innervate the levator palpebrae superioris, which is responsible for lifting the upper eyelid.

The Edinger-Westphal nucleus is the parasympathetic nucleus of the oculomotor nerve and is situated just dorsal to the motor nucleus (Figure 2). Preganglionic fibers leave it, join the voluntary motor fibers, and pass out to the orbit. There the parasympathetic fibers separate and most of them terminate in the ciliary ganglion (Figure 2). Here they synapse with postganglionic fibers that stimulate the sphincter pupillae muscle, causing the pupil to constrict. A few of the preganglionic fibers pass through the ciliary ganglion and end on the episcleral ganglion, where they synapse with postganglionic fibers that innervate the ciliary muscle that is concerned with lens accommodation for near vision.

Clinical Aspects

Since the oculomotor nucleus receives a bilateral upper motor neuron supply via the corticobulbar tract (Chapter 8), one rarely sees an upper motor (a supranuclear) lesion that affects this nerve. However, if the oculomotor nerve is damaged, there is a lower motor neuron paralysis of the muscles it supplies, and the eyeball is pulled laterally and downward by the unopposed lateral rectus muscle (supplied by the abducens nerve) and the superior oblique muscle (supplied by the trochlear). Because the levator palpebrae is paralyzed, the upper eyelid droops — a condition known as "ptosis." In addition, the parasympathetic fibers will also be damaged and, as a result, the sphincter pupillae will be paralyzed. The dilator pupillae, supplied by the sympathetics, is now unopposed; consequently the pupil is widely dilated and cannot constrict (in other words, there is a "fixed pupil"). Also, oculomotor nerve damage causes difficulty in visual accommodation because the ciliary muscle is paralyzed.

THE TRIGEMINAL NERVE (V)

This trigeminal nerve has general sensory fibers as well as voluntary motor neurons. The sensory fibers (Chapter 6) convey general sensations of pain, temperature, touch, pressure, and proprioception from the face, cornea, mouth, nasal activities, sinuses, tongue, teeth, meninges, outer surface of the eardrum, and temperomandibular joint. The motor component consists of voluntary or lower motor neurons that supply the four muscles of mastication, i.e., the temporalis, the digastric, the lateral, and the medial pterygoids (Figure 1c). In addition, the trigeminal motor fibers innervate the anterior belly of the digastric, the mylohyoid and the tensor tympani and tensor veli palatini muscles. The motor nucleus of the trigeminal nerve is located in the pons near the main sensory nucleus.

Clinical Aspects

If the entire nerve is cut or damaged there will be a complete loss of sensation in the facial area on the same side, as well as difficulty in chewing, speaking, and so on. Because this nerve also receives a bilateral innervation from the cerebral cortex, one rarely sees cases of upper motor neuron lesions (see also "Clinical Aspects" in Chapter 6).

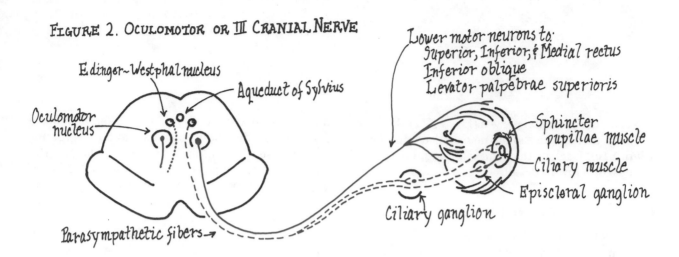

FIGURE 2. OCULOMOTOR OR III CRANIAL NERVE

Edinger-Westphal nucleus

Aqueduct of Sylvius

Oculomotor nucleus

Lower motor neurons to:
Superior, Inferior, & Medial rectus
Inferior oblique
Levator palpebrae superioris

Sphincter pupillae muscle

Ciliary muscle

Episcleral ganglion

Ciliary ganglion

Parasympathetic fibers

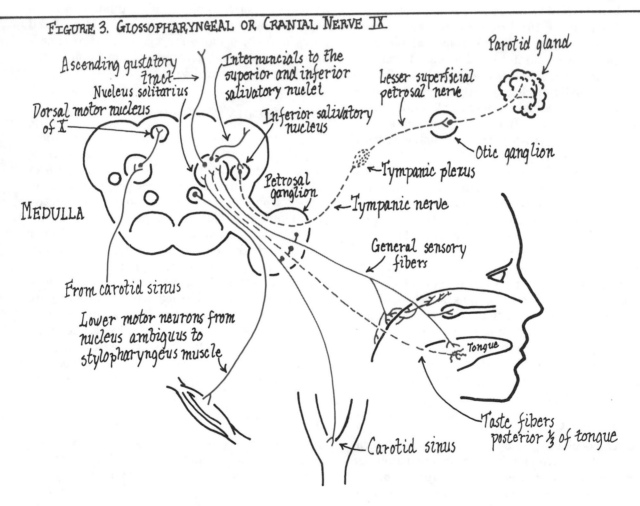

FIGURE 3. GLOSSOPHARYNGEAL OR CRANIAL NERVE IX

Ascending gustatory tract

Nucleus solitarius

Dorsal motor nucleus of X

Internuncials to the superior and inferior salivatory nuclei

Inferior salivatory nucleus

Lesser superficial petrosal nerve

Parotid gland

Otic ganglion

Tympanic plexus

Petrosal ganglion

Tympanic nerve

MEDULLA

General sensory fibers

From carotid sinus

Lower motor neurons from nucleus ambiguus to stylopharyngeus muscle

Tongue

Carotid sinus

Taste fibers posterior ⅓ of tongue

PLATE 13~2.

THE FACIAL NERVE (VII)

The facial nerve is a more complex nerve that has three major components:

1. Special sensory fibers for taste from the anterior two-thirds of the tongue
2. Parasympathetic fibers to the sublingual, submaxillary, and lacrimal glands
3. Voluntary motor fibers to all the muscles of facial expression

The taste receptors are located on the anterior two-thirds of the tongue, and their fibers pass back to the brainstem (Figure 4). In their course, they merge with the lingual branch of the trigeminal nerve, but then they separate from it to form the nerve known as the *chorda tympani*. This nerve enters the skull through a small fissure and passes into the temporal bone, in which is situated the geniculate ganglion. Here are located the cell bodies of the taste neurons, whose axons pass into the pons and end in the nucleus solitarius (Figures 4 and 4a). From this nucleus 2° ascending gustatory tracts arise that reach conscious levels; however, their exact course is unknown. In addition, there are reflex pathways for taste sensations. For example, when one tastes something pleasant there is a reflex salivation, and this pathway involves the parasympathetic component of the seventh as well as the ninth cranial nerve. From the nucleus ambiguus, internuncials pass down to the superior salivatory nucleus and synapse with preganglionic neurons (Figure 4). Their axons leave the pons, enter the internal auditory meatus and travel through the geniculate ganglion. They then separate from the rest of the facial nerve fibers to form the chorda tympani, which merges with the lingual nerve. After "hitching a ride" with the lingual nerve, the preganglionic parasympathetics again separate and terminate in the submaxillary ganglion. Here they synapse with the postganglionic neurons, which stimulate the submaxillary and sublingual salivary glands. Other preganglionic parasympathetic fibers from the superior salivatory nucleus follow a different course and reach the sphenopalatine ganglion, where they synapse with postganglionic neurons (Figure 4). These postganglionic neurons follow a complicated pathway to reach the lacrimal gland and the mucus-secreting cells of the nose and mouth (Figure 4).

The last major component of the facial nerve is voluntary motor fibers to all the muscles of facial expression. Their nucleus is found in the tegmentum of the pons below the nucleus of cranial nerve VI (Figure 4). The emerging motor fibers pass up and loop around the abducens nucleus, causing a bulge on the floor of the fourth ventricle that is known as the *facial colliculus*. These motor fibers then join the rest of the components and enter the internal auditory meatus. After the taste and parasympathetic neurons have separated from the main bundle, the remaining voluntary motor fibers leave the skull at the stylomastoid foramen, separate into five main branches that supply all the muscles of facial expression, as well as the posterior belly of the digastric and the mylohyoid muscles. Within the temporal bone some motor fibers supply the stapedius muscle of the middle ear, which acts as a "brake" on the hearing apparatus and prevents hyperacoustica.

Clinical Aspects

One of the most common pathological conditions involving the seventh nerve is Bell's palsy. In this condition nerve damage of unknown etiology results in a characteristic lower motor neuron paralysis of all the muscles of the facial expression on the affected side. The person is unable to close the affected eye because the orbicularis occuli muscle is paralyzed and the consequently unopposed muscles on the unaffected side contract and pull the mouth up in a characteristic grin. The lesion may affect the stapedius muscle, and the patient will also suffer from hyperacoustica. In addition there may be a partial loss of taste, salivation, and lacrimation.

Since the lower part of the motor nucleus receives its upper motor neuron supply only from the contralateral corticobulbar tract (Chapter 8), an upper motor or supranuclear lesion will produce a contralateral spastic paralysis of the muscles in the lower half of the face. Because the muscles of the upper half of the face have a bilateral nerve supply, the patient with such a lesion can still close his eye and wrinkle his brow. These two actions help differentiate between Bell's palsy, which is a lower motor neuron paralysis, and an upper motor neuron lesion.

THE GLOSSOPHARYNGEAL NERVE (IX)

The glossopharyngeal nerve also has three major components:

1. Special sensory taste neurons, from the posterior third of the tongue
2. Parasympathetic fibers to the parotid gland

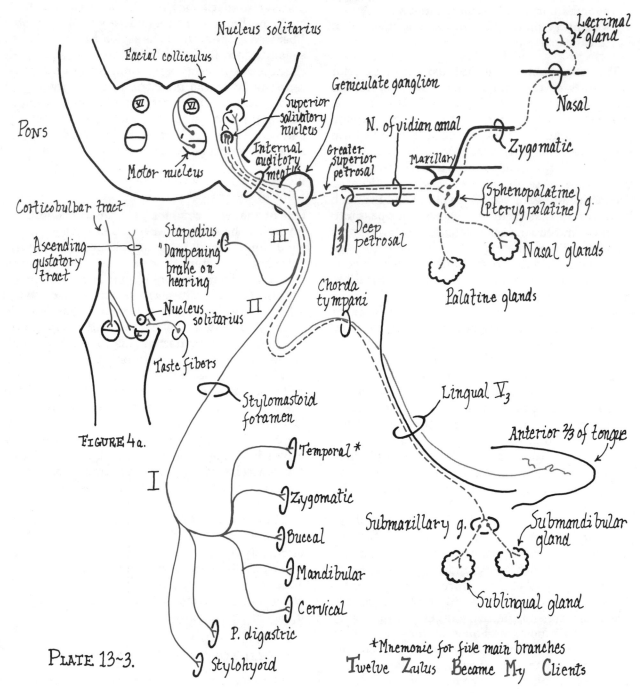

FIGURE 4. THE FACIAL OR VII CRANIAL NERVE

Nucleus solitarius

Facial colliculus

Lacrimal gland

Nasal

Geniculate ganglion

Superior salivatory nucleus

N. of vidian canal

Zygomatic

Pons

Maxillary

Motor nucleus

Internal auditory meatus

Greater superior petrosal

(Sphenopalatine) (Pterygpalatine) g.

Corticobulbar tract

Deep petrosal

Nasal glands

Ascending gustatory tract

Stapedius "Dampening" brake on hearing

III

Palatine glands

Chorda tympani

Nucleus solitarius

II

Taste fibers

Lingual V₃

Anterior ⅔ of tongue

FIGURE 4a.

Stylomastoid foramen

I

Temporal *

Zygomatic

Buccal

Mandibular

Submaxillary g.

Submandibular gland

Cervical

P. digastric

Sublingual gland

PLATE 13~3.

Stylohyoid

*Mnemonic for five main branches
Twelve Zulus Became My Clients

3. General sensory neurons from the auditory tube, the inner surface of the tympanic membrane, the pharynx, and the carotid sinus

On the surface of the posterior one-third of the tongue are situated the taste receptors of the ninth cranial nerve. The cell bodies of these neurons are located in the petrosal ganglion (Figure 3) and their axons end in the nucleus solitarius, which extends down from the pons into the medulla. Here they synapse with ascending gustatory fibers that eventually reach conscious levels, but their pathway and final cortical localization are unclear. As is the case with the seventh nerve, there are also reflex arcs involving taste. From the solitarius nucleus, short internuncials pass to the inferior salivatory nucleus and synapse with preganglionic parasympathetic neurons. The axons of the latter leave the medulla along with the other glossopharyngeal fibers but then separate and follow a long course (Figure 3) to reach the otic ganglion. Here they synapse with postganglionic parasympathetic neurons that stimulate the parotid salivatory gland. Other internuncials from the nucleus solitarius pass up and synapse in the superior salivatory nucleus, whose fibers reach the sublingual and submaxillary gland (see the discussion of the facial nerve above).

The last major component of the glossopharyngeal nerve is the general sensory component, involving pain, pressure, touch, and temperature. The receptors are found in the Eustachian tube, the middle ear, the inner surface of the tympanic membrane, the uvula, the carotid sinus, and the nasal and oval pharynx. The fibers from these areas pass back to the petrosal ganglia, which "houses" their cell bodies, and terminate in the nucleus solitarius. Here they synapse with neurons of various tracts, e.g., some that ascend to consciousness and others that set off important reflexes, such as the 'gag' reflex (see Clinical Aspects). Another example involves the carotid sinus, which is sensitive to blood pressure changes; when blood pressure rises it stimulates this receptor, which "fires off" a compensatory reflex. From the nucleus solitarius an internuncial neuron passes to the dorsal motor nucleus of the vagus nerve (cranial nerve X) and synapses with a parasympathetic neuron. The latter descends to the heart and stimulates it to slow down the heart rate, thus lowering the blood pressure.

The glossopharyngeal nerve also has voluntary motor neurons that stimulate the stylopharyngeus muscle (Figure 3).

Clinical Aspects

If the uvula or oral pharynx is touched, a "gag" reflex is set off and the trachea is closed by the epiglottis. However, when a patient is under general gas anesthesia, this reflex does not work. Furthermore, the unconscious patient often vomits. It is therefore *absolutely imperative* that, before general surgery, *no food or liquid be given* to the patient 12 hours before the procedure: otherwise the patient may vomit while unconscious and the acid contents from the stomach will enter the now wide-open trachea and lungs — with a fatal result.

THE VAGUS NERVE (X)

The vagus nerve, a vital nerve, has two major components:
1. Parasympathetic fibers to all the autonomic structures of the chest and abdomen up to the left colic flexure (Chapter 12, Figure 3)
2. Voluntary motor fibers to the muscles of larynx and pharynx involved in talking and swallowing

The vagus also has sensory fibers from the viscera, the carotid body (a chemoreceptor), the dura of the posterior cranial fossa, and the lower part of the pharynx. The cell bodies are located in the jugular and nodose ganglia and the axons end in the nucleus solitarius (Figure 1c).

The parasympathetic fibers arise from the dorsal motor nucleus of the vagus nerve, which is found in the floor of the fourth ventricle of the medulla, just lateral to the hypoglossal nucleus (Atlas, Figure 14). The preganglionic fibers leave and descend into the chest and abdomen, where they synapse in ganglia that are situated on or in the organs that are innervated (Figure 1c of this chapter and Chapter 12, Figure 3).

The motor fibers arise in the nucleus ambiguus of the medulla (Figure 1c and Atlas, Figure 14) and leave the brainstem with the parasympathetic fibers. They soon branch away from the vagus and supply all the muscles of the larynx and most of those in the pharynx. Damage to these motor fibers or their nucleus results in a lower motor neuron paralysis, with difficulty in talking or swallowing.

Chapter 14

THE AUDITORY PATHWAY

The eighth cranial nerve, the acoustovestibular (vestibulocochlear), is entirely sensory and has two important parts: the acoustic part, which transmits sound impulses from the ear to the brain, and the vestibular part, which is concerned with maintaining body equilibrium. This chapter deals with the acoustic division, which is basically very simple.

In the cochlear apparatus of the inner ear are situated specialized receptors — the *hair cells* — which are stimulated by auditory vibrations from the external and middle ear. In the cochlea these hair cells synapse with primary neurons, the cell bodies of which are localized in the spiral ganglia that's also situated in the cochlea (Figure 1). From here axons pass to the brainstem, enter it at the pontomedullary junction, and immediately bifurcate, with one branch terminating in the *dorsal cochlear nucleus* and the other in the *ventral cochlear nucleus* (Figure 1). From the dorsal cochlear nucleus some secondary axons cross over to the other side and ascend to reach the nucleus of the inferior colliculus. Others don't cross, but ascend ipsilaterally and also terminate in the nucleus of the inferior colliculus (Figure 1). These ascending crossed and uncrossed fibers comprise the *lateral lemniscus.*

Most of the axons from the ventral cochlear nucleus decussate and pass up in the lateral lemniscus to end in the nucleus of the inferior colliculus. A few don't cross over but ascend in the ipsilateral lateral lemniscus (Figure 1). Thus, both the dorsal and the ventral cochlear nucleus send out crossed and uncrossed fibers to the nucleus of the inferior colliculus. From here fibers are relayed out, via the brachium of the inferior colliculus, to the medial geniculate body that lies adjacent to the superior colliculus. In this body they synapse with neurons, the axons of which form the auditory radiations that end in the 1° auditory cortex of the superior temporal gyrus — also known as areas 41 and 42 — the hearing center.

ACCESSORY DETAILS AND CLINICAL ASPECTS

1. The decussating axons from the dorsal and ventral cochlear nuclei form a large distinct mass, the *trapezoid body* (Figure 1).
2. The right and left nuclei of the inferior colliculus are connected to each other by commissural neurons (Figure 1).
3. Some of the fibers in the lateral lemniscus don't end in the nucleus of the inferior colliculus but pass straight up to the medial geniculate body (Figure 1).
4. On the other hand, many axons from the dorsal and ventral cochlear nuclei don't ascend directly to the midbrain, but make many synaptic stops along the way. For example, crossed fibers from both nuclei synapse in the superior olivary nucleus, which then relays up to the higher areas (Figure 2). This is not important clinically. What is important is the fact that each auditory cortex receives fibers from the left and right cochlear nuclei, or, put another way, the cochlear nuclei of the right side pro-

FIGURE 1

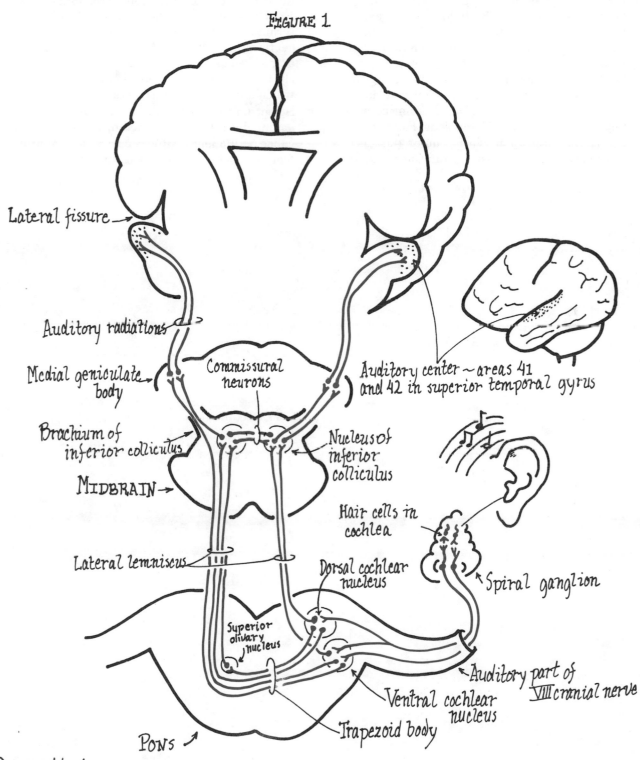

Lateral fissure

Auditory radiations

Medial geniculate body

Commissural neurons

Auditory center ~ areas 41 and 42 in superior temporal gyrus

Brachium of inferior colliculus

Nucleus of inferior colliculus

MIDBRAIN

Hair cells in cochlea

Lateral lemniscus

Dorsal cochlear nucleus

Spiral ganglion

Superior olivary nucleus

Auditory part of VIII cranial nerve

Ventral cochlear nucleus

Trapezoid body

PONS

PLATE 14~1.

ject onto the left and right auditory cortex, and left cochlear nuclei project to both hearing centers. The clinical significance of this bilateral representation is obvious. If, for example, the right auditory cortex is damaged, then the patient will still hear from both ears, using the intact left auditory cortex. This holds true for damage at other sites along the central pathway, i.e., right medial geniculate body, the right nucleus of the inferior colliculus, or the right lateral lemniscus. However, if the right auditory nerve is cut or damaged anywhere along its path — from the ear up to and including the cochlear nuclei — then the person will be deaf in the right ear, and what holds true for the right side is true for the left.

5. From the nucleus of the inferior colliculus, internuncial axons pass out to various motor centers to mediate auditory reflexes. For example, when one hears a sudden loud noise, the eyes close and the body "jumps," both of which are reactions of the startle reflex.

6. Streptomycin, when given in massive, life-saving doses to combat meningitis, may often cause permanent deafness as a serious side effect because it damages the auditory nerve.

Chapter 15

VISUAL PATHWAYS AND OPTIC REFLEXES

The visual pathways are among the more important pathways of the nervous system. Because injuries to them are common, the physician must know and understand them "cold."

Light rays from an object in the visual field enter the eyeball, are inverted by the lens, and strike the nervous layer, the *retina*. The retina is composed of several layers and types of neurons, among them being the light-sensitive *rods* and *cones*. Each eye has a temporal and a nasal visual field, and, because of the inversion by the lens, the temporal visual field is projected onto the nasal retinal field and the nasal visual field falls on the temporal retinal field (Figure 1). Loss of vision is always described with reference to the visual fields, not the retinal fields. These concepts can be quite confusing at first, and it pays the student to read and review each concept slowly and attentively.

Axons from nerve cells in the eye pass posteriorly in the optic nerve. At the chiasma, those from the nasal retinal field cross over to join the axons from the temporal retinal field, which don't cross (Figure 1). Together they continue posteriorly in the optic tract and end in the lateral geniculate body of the diencephalon. Here they synapse with neurons that sweep out to form the optic radiations, which end in the visual cortex of the occipital lobe. This cortex begins at the occipital pole and is situated on the *cuneate* and *lingual gyri*, which border on the *calcarine fissure* (Figures 1 and 2). Thus, the left visual field of each eye is represented on the right occipital cortex, while the right visual fields are represented on the left occipital cortex (Figure 1). The lens also inverts the upper visual field onto the lower part of the retina and vice versa (Figure 2). This pattern is maintained throughout the pathway, so that the cuneate gyrus, which is above the calcarine fissure, receives impulses from the lower visual field, and the lingual gyrus, which is below the fissure, gets impulses from the upper visual field (Figure 2). Finally, the *macula* — the central area of the retina where vision is the sharpest — sends its impulses to the occipital poles (Figure 1).

CLINICAL ASPECTS

In an eye examination, the fields of vision of each eye are tested and mapped out. If, for example, the right optic nerve is damaged (Example 1), both fields of vision of that eye are affected — in short, *anopsia* or *blindness* of the right eye results.

Example 2 illustrates how an *aneurism* of the right carotid artery, which lies adjacent to the lateral part of the optic chiasma, can interfere with the temporal axons from the right retina, thus producing *hemianopsia* (half blindness) in the right eye. Since the visual field affected is the nasal field, we speak of a nasal hemianopsia of the right eye, or right nasal hemianopsia.

Example 3 shows how the pituitary gland, lying between the optic tracts near the chiasma, can develop an expanding tumor that presses on the decussating nasal axons. This can produce hemianopsia in the temporal visual fields of both eyes — a *bitemporal hemianopsia*.

Examples 4, 5, and 6 illustrate how a lesion in the right optic tract, the right optic radiations, or the right visual cortex can produce loss of vision in the left visual fields of both eyes, which is called a *left homonymous hemianopsia*.

Because the visual field of each eye is divided into nasal and temporal parts plus upper and lower parts, the term 'quadrant' is often used: e.g., upper quadrant or lower right quadrant, etc. There can also be various quadratic anopsias.

OPTIC REFLEXES

If light from a small source, e.g., a pencil flashlight, is shone into one eye from a close distance, there will be pupillary reflex constriction in both

OPTIC PATHWAYS

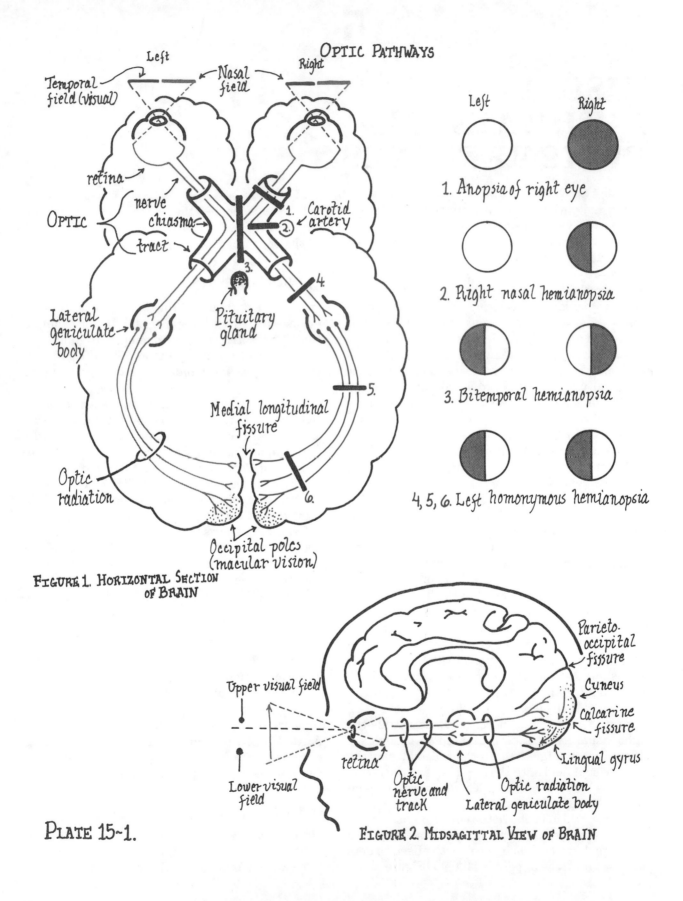

Left — Temporal field (visual) — Nasal field — Right

retina

OPTIC nerve chiasma — tract

Carotid artery

1.

2.

3.

4.

Lateral geniculate body

Pituitary gland

5.

Medial longitudinal fissure

6.

Optic radiation

Occipital poles (macular vision)

FIGURE 1. HORIZONTAL SECTION OF BRAIN

Left   Right

1. Anopsia of right eye

2. Right nasal hemianopsia

3. Bitemporal hemianopsia

4, 5, 6. Left homonymous hemianopsia

Upper visual field

Lower visual field

retina

Optic nerve and track

Lateral geniculate body

Optic radiation

Parieto-occipital fissure

Cuneus

Calcarine fissure

Lingual gyrus

PLATE 15~1.

FIGURE 2. MIDSAGITTAL VIEW OF BRAIN

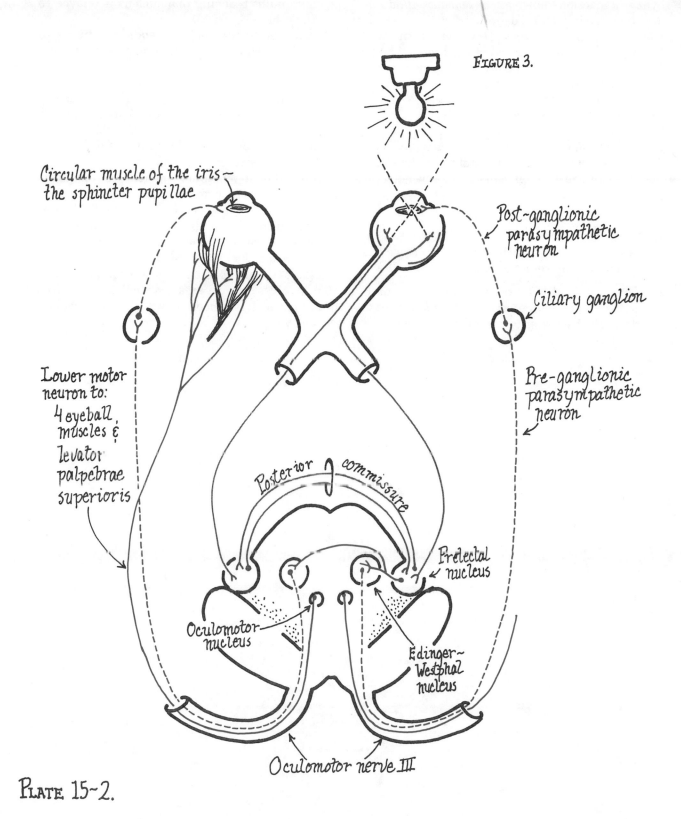

FIGURE 3.

Circular muscle of the iris —
the sphincter pupillae

Post-ganglionic
parasympathetic
neuron

Ciliary ganglion

Lower motor
neuron to:
4 eyeball
muscles &
levator
palpebrae
superioris

Pre-ganglionic
parasympathetic
neuron

Posterior commissure

Prelectal
nucleus

Oculomotor
nucleus

Edinger-
Westphal
nucleus

Oculomotor nerve III

PLATE 15~2.

eyes — a reaction known as *consensual validation.* As you have just learned, optic tract fibers end in the lateral geniculate body. However, about 1% of them peel off just before reaching the geniculate body and terminate in the pretectal nucleus of the midbrain (Figure 3). From here internuncial fibers pass to the parasympathetic Edinger-Westphal nucleus, which then automatically discharges motor stimuli to the circular muscle of the iris, causing pupillary constriction (Figure 3). Therefore, there are three ways that light impulses from one eye can cause reflex constriction in both pupils:

1. Some optic fibers, from the right eye's nasal retinal field, cross in the chiasma to reach the contralateral pretectal nucleus (Figure 3).

2. The right and left pretectal nuclei are interconnected by commissural neurons that pass through the posterior commissure. Therefore,

a stimulus reaching one nucleus is relayed to the other (Figure 3).

3. Each pretectal nucleus sends out fibers to both the right and left Edinger-Westphal nucleus (Figure 3).

The pupillary light reflex is one of the most useful and important reflexes in medical practice. It occurs even when a person is unconscious; if it can't be elicited, a serious condition in the CNS, especially the brainstem, is indicated.

The Edinger-Westphal nucleus is also concerned with the accommodation reflex, whereby the lens of the eye accommodates itself for near and far vision. From this nucleus, motor stimuli are sent out over the pre- and postganglionic fibers to reach the ciliary muscle that controls the AP diameter of the lens. This is a complex reflex that involves cortical areas as well as the *nucleus of Perla,* which is concerned with the convergence of the eyes.

Chapter 16

THE OLFACTORY SYSTEM

Many lower animal forms, such as dogs, deer, amphibians, and certain birds, depend primarily on the sense of smell to locate food, to distinguish friend from foe, and to attract the opposite sex. Consequently, the olfactory system is very highly developed in these animals and is closely connected to the aggressive drive, since this drive is necessary to obtain the above-mentioned objects. In humans, the sense of smell is probably the least important of the major senses, but its pathways, carried over from lower forms, are the most complex of the nervous system. Furthermore, there is a great deal of contradictory data, based on experiments in animals, and the beginning student who opens most "neuro" texts finds himself immersed in a welter of conflicting theories couched in the most obtuse and strange terminology. (It is a rule of thumb in science, medicine, and other subjects that, the more theories and the more terminology there are concerning a subject, then the less is known about it, and psychology and psychoanalysis are excellent examples of this.) This chapter discusses the basic, generally agreed upon facts concerning the olfactory system, and touches very lightly on the experimental data.

In the epithelial tissue of the nasal cavity are located receptor cells sensitive to smell. These 1° neurons, which are bipolar, pass up into the olfactory bulb, where they synapse with 2° neurons whose axons form the olfactory tract, which runs posteriorly and then bifurcates into a lateral and medial olfactory tract, or *stria* (Figures 1 and 2).

(The area between the bifurcating stria forms the anterior perforated area (Figure 2).) The axons of the medial olfactory stria terminate in the paraolfactory, or septal, area and the anterior perforated area, while some enter the anterior commissure and cross over to terminate in the contralateral septal area (Figures 1 and 2). The fibers of the lateral olfactory stria end in the cortex of the uncus and in the underlying amygdaloid nucleus (Figures 1 and 2). It is believed that the septal area, the anterior perforated substance, and the cortex of the uncus are the cerebral areas concerned with the "interpretation" of smell.

In humans the sense of smell can trigger various emotions and their related reflexes. For example, the smell of good food causes pleasure and salivation, while that of rotten eggs causes disgust, nausea, and even vomiting. An enticing perfume may result in sexual arousal (isn't that its basic purpose?), while other odors may elicit long-forgotten memories. The major reflex pathways are as follows: From the amygdaloid nucleus, fibers collect in a bundle, the *stria terminalis,* which loops around and terminates in the hypothalamus (Figure 3). The amygdala also sends short fibers to the adjacent hippocampus, where they synapse with neurons that form a large bundle, the *fornix.* This distinctive tract curves up and around to end in the mamillary bodies of the hypothalamus (Figure 3). Finally, from the septal or paraolfactory area, short fibers pass to terminate also in the hypothalamus (Figure 3). (It isn't surprising that all

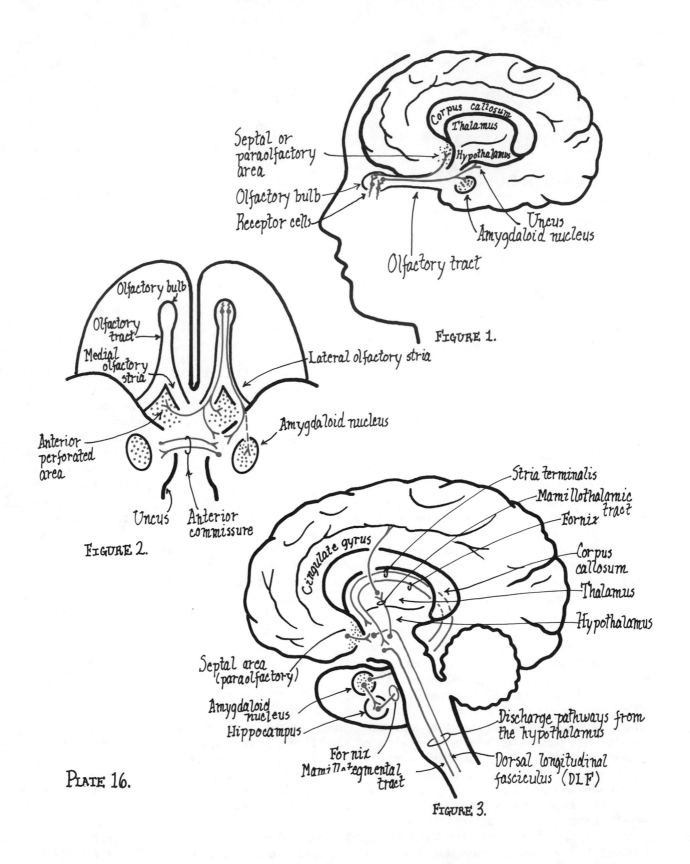

Septal or paraolfactory area

Olfactory bulb

Receptor cells

Corpus callosum

Thalamus

Hypothalamus

Uncus

Amygdaloid nucleus

Olfactory tract

FIGURE 1.

Olfactory bulb

Olfactory tract

Medial olfactory stria

Lateral olfactory stria

Amygdaloid nucleus

Anterior perforated area

Uncus

Anterior commissure

FIGURE 2.

Stria terminalis

Mamillothalamic tract

Fornix

Corpus callosum

Thalamus

Hypothalamus

Cingulate gyrus

Septal area (paraolfactory)

Amygdaloid nucleus

Hippocampus

Fornix

Mamillotegmental tract

Discharge pathways from the hypothalamus

Dorsal longitudinal fasciculus (DLF)

FIGURE 3.

PLATE 16.

these reflex pathways end in the hypothalamus, for, as shown in the following chapter, this is the main coordination and reflex-discharge center for many sensations, such as smell, taste, and emotions, as well as the control center of the autonomic nervous system.) Reflex-discharge pathways carry smell sensations from the hypothalamus to the appropriate motor nuclei and reticular areas in the brainstem. The two main tracts are the mamillotegmental and the dorsal longitudinal fasciculus (Figure 3). Finally, from the mamillary bodies there is a large bundle, the mamillothalamic tract, which ends in the anterior group of the thalamic nuclei, and from here the impulses are relayed to the cingulate gyrus (Figure 3). In spite of much experimental work, no functional significance of this pathway has been discovered.

CLINICAL ASPECTS

Loss of smell results from damage to the receptor cells, the olfactory bulb, or the olfactory tract, and is known medically as *anosmia*. Lesions of the temporal lobe in the area of the uncus and the amygdala often produce olfactory hallucinations, epileptic seizures, or a combination of both, known as *uncinate fits* when the epileptic fit is preceded by olfactory aura.

In monkeys the removal of the amygdala results in very docile, somnolent animals, while in cats the same procedure produces animals who are very aggressive in unprovoked situations — a condition known as sham rage. However, in both species the procedure causes a greatly increased sexual drive.

Chapter 17

THE RETICULAR SYSTEM

The reticular system is a phylogenetically old system that is divided anatomically and physiologically into two parts: a descending and an ascending formation.

DESCENDING RETICULAR FORMATION

The descending reticular formation is a system concerned with:

1. Relaying impulses from the hypothalamus to various target organs of the autonomic nervous system.
2. Relaying involuntary motor impulses from the extrapyramidal systems to voluntary muscles.

Scattered deep in the brainstem are the groups of diffuse nuclei or areas (some authors and investigators call them formations) belonging to this system. In the midbrain they are called the *deep* and *dorsal tegmental nuclei;* in the pons they are called the *central tegmental nucleus;* and in the medulla they are the *central* and *inferior nuclei.* Some books also mention other descending reticular nuclei or call them by different names, but the main point to grasp is not the exact number of nuclei but the fact that they exist and their function.

These nuclei or formations receive stimuli from the hypothalamus fiber tracts, such as the dorsal longitudinal fasciculus and the mamillotegmental tract (Figure 1). In addition, various basal ganglia, such as the globus pallidus, substantia nigra, and the subthalamic nucleus, project fibers that terminate in these nuclei. Lastly, the vestibular system, which is also extrapyramidal, sends some of its fibers to the reticular nuclei (see the chapters on the vestibular and cerebellar systems).

These incoming fibers synapse with neurons whose axons then leave the reticular nuclei and form the lateral and medial reticulospinal tracts. These are descending, crossed and uncrossed, multisynaptic pathways that travel down to all levels of the spinal cord in the lateral and ventral white columns. In the cord they synapse either on the ventral horn cells, which form the final common pathway, or on the preganglionic neurons in the intermediate gray horn.

ASCENDING RETICULAR FORMATION

The ascending reticular formation, better known as the reticular activating system, is concerned with degrees of conscious alertness as well as with sleep. Situated in the medulla, pons, and midbrain, i.e., the brainstem, are groups of poorly defined nuclei that are connected to each other by a chain of multisynaptic neurons. Because the nuclei and their interconnecting chain have a diffuse and poorly defined appearance, they were given the name *reticular system.*

All the major sensory pathways (e.g., the spinothalamic, for pain, temperature, touch, and pressure; the auditory, the visual, etc.) send collateral axons that end in the nuclei of the reticular activating system. These nuclei then send the sensory stimuli they have received up the multisynaptic chain, which ends primarily in a group of nuclei of the thalamus known as the midline group. As has already been shown, the thalamus serves as a relay center for many sensory pathways — as well as motor ones — and it is not surprising that it also serves as a relay for the reticular activating system. From the thalamic midline, nuclei impulses are relayed up to the cerebral cortex*, where they influence states of mental alertness and sleep. What exactly do we mean by this statement? Sleeping animals and humans exhibit a characteristic electroencephalogram (EEG) wave pattern, but if the reticular activating nuclei of sleeping animals are experimentally stimulated, the animals awaken, and we see that the change

---

*Exactly how these impulses are relayed and what specific regions of the cerebral cortex they reach are not known.

FIGURE 1. SCHEMATIC DIAGRAM OF THE DESCENDING RETICULAR FORMATION

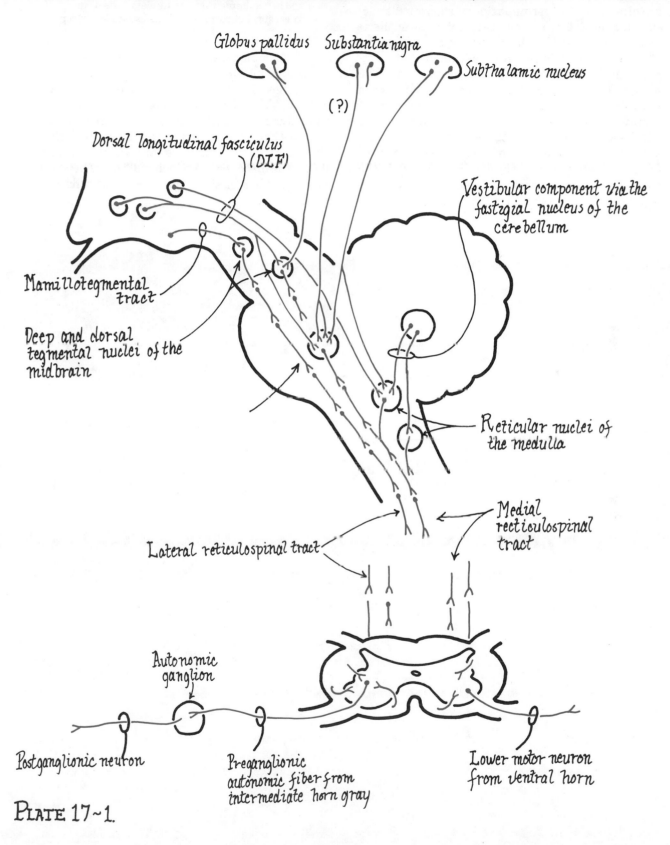

Globus pallidus

Substantia nigra

Subthalamic nucleus

(?)

Dorsal longitudinal fasciculus (DLF)

Vestibular component via the fastigial nucleus of the cerebellum

Mamillotegmental tract

Deep and dorsal tegmental nuclei of the midbrain

Reticular nuclei of the medulla

Lateral reticulospinal tract

Medial reticulospinal tract

Autonomic ganglion

Postganglionic neuron

Preganglionic autonomic fiber from intermediate horn gray

Lower motor neuron from ventral horn

PLATE 17~1.

from sleep to wakefulness is accompanied by a change in the EEG wave pattern. In animals that are already awake, stimulation of the reticular activating nuclei produces states of greater alertness accompanied by characteristic changes in the EEG pattern. It is therefore assumed that alertness and/or sleep is largely dependent on the amount of stimuli reaching the cerebral cortex via the reticular activating system. If the amount of stimuli from the outside world is reduced, there will be a lowering of alertness, and sleep may result. On the other hand, an increase in the amount of stimulation reaching the cerebral cortex via the ascending reticular formation results in greater alertness. In a nutshell, we may say that:

↓ stimulation from various sensory systems into the reticular nuclei → ↓ amount of stimulation to the thalamic midline nuclei → ↓ stimulus to cerebral cortex → ↓ alertness and/or sleep

This simple outline is just one aspect of an extremely complex picture, most of which is still unrevealed to us. One should not conclude that sleep or alertness is totally dependent on the state of the reticular activating system; there are many other factors — e.g., metabolic and psychic factors — that play a part in alertness and sleep. There are also many factors that we know nothing about, the discovery of which will throw new light on the problem of sleep, alertness, and consciousness.

Chapter **18**

THE HYPOTHALAMUS

The hypothalamus is one of the smallest areas of the brain, yet no other region has so many different and vital functions. As its name indicates, it lies beneath the thalamus: it is seen well in a midsagittal section (Figures 3 and 4 in the Atlas), where it extends from the lamina terminalis to the midbrain. Separating it from the overlying thalamus is a shallow groove, the *hypothalamic sulcus*. The hypothalamus thus forms the lateral wall of the lower part of the third ventricle and is also seen in cross-sections (Figure 6 in the Atlas). If one looks at the base of the brain, the hypothalamus forms the area that lies posterior to the optic chiasma and includes the infundibulum and mamillary bodies. Packed into this small region are many nuclei and areas (Figure 1) that are concerned with such functions as temperature control, sleep, water metabolism, secretion of hormones, control of blood pressure, hunger, and maintaining a balance between the sympathetic and parasympathetic divisions. It also plays a part in emotional reactions and possibly other situations.

HEAT REGULATION

The anterior hypothalamic area is concerned with heat regulation of the body. When there is an increase in body temperature, the heated blood passes through the anterior hypothalamic area and sets off a mechanism that facilitates heat loss (Figure 2). Fibers leave the anterior hypothalamic area and join the dorsal longitudinal fasciculus (DLF), which is the major descending pathway from the hypothalamus. The DLF terminates in the descending reticular nuclei of the brainstem, where it synapses with neurons of the medial and lateral reticulospinal tracts. These then descend the cord and stimulate the sympathetic nervous system and voluntary muscles. Other fibers of the DLF terminate in, and stimulate, the cardiac and respiratory centers in the medulla. The results of

all these stimuli are the following reactions, which serve to reduce body temperature:

1. Dilation of peripheral blood vessels beneath the skin, with a subsequent increase in heat radiation.
2. An increase in sweating, which reduces heat. (Evaporation is a cooling process.)
3. Increase in respiratory rate, with "blowing off" of hot air from the lungs.
4. A decrease in the body's metabolic rate.
5. Increases in peripheral blood flow accompanied by increased heat dissipation.

If we experimentally destroy an animal's anterior hypothalamic region, it is unable to respond to heat increases of its environment. Thus, when the temperature rises its body temperature rises, and eventually it will die from heat prostration.

Cold regulation is controlled by the posterior hypothalamic area. When the temperature of the environment drops, the body becomes cooler. The cooled blood passes through the posterior hypothalamic area (Figure 2) and sets off a mechanism that is just the opposite of the one just discussed. The pathways are basically the same, e.g., DLF, reticular nuclei, and reticulospinal tracts. The reactions set off to conserve body heat are as follows:

1. Peripheral vasoconstriction, with a subsequent decrease in the amount of heat lost by radiation.
2. A decrease in peripheral blood flow.
3. An increase in body metabolism.
4. Shivering of voluntary muscles. Shivering is work in which energy, in the form of heat, is produced. (There is, of course, also energy of motion.)
5. A decrease in the respiratory rate.

Experimental lesions in the posterior hypothalamic area produce animals that are unable to adjust to cold environments, and their bodies become as cold as the surroundings.

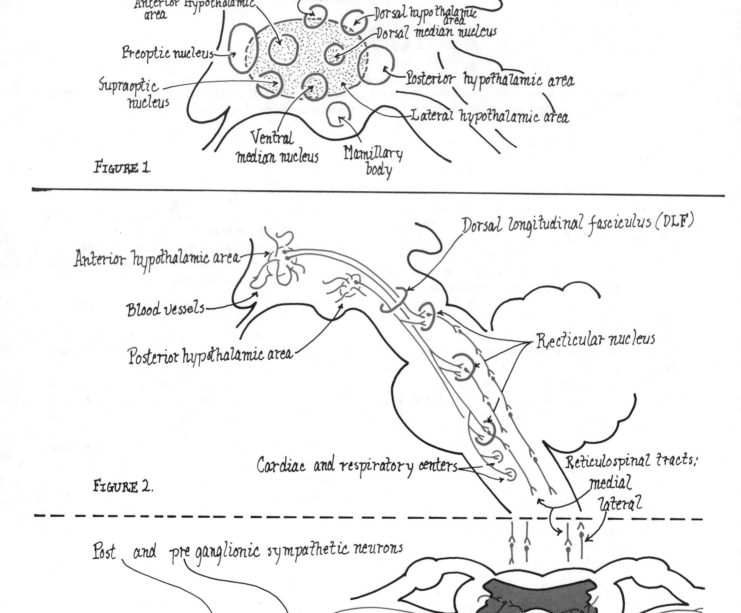

FIGURE 1.

Anterior Hypothalamic area
Paraventral nucleus
Dorsal hypothalamic area
Dorsal median nucleus
Preoptic nucleus
Supraoptic nucleus
Posterior hypothalamic area
Lateral hypothalamic area
Ventral median nucleus
Mamillary body

FIGURE 2.

Dorsal longitudinal fasciculus (DLF)
Anterior hypothalamic area
Blood vessels
Posterior hypothalamic area
Recticular nucleus
Cardiac and respiratory centers
Reticulospinal tracts; medial lateral

Post and pre ganglionic sympathetic neurons
Intermediate horn gray
Ventral horn gray
Lower motor neuron

PLATE 18~1.

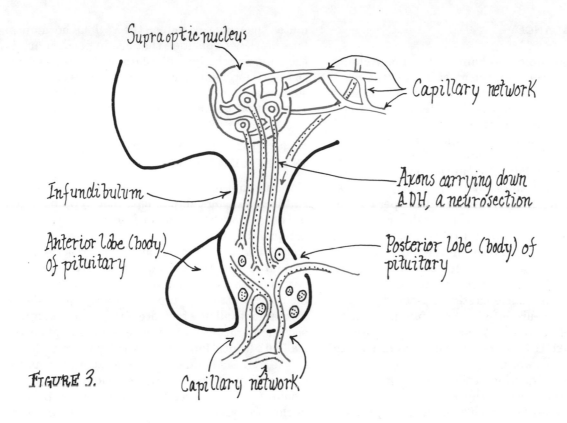

Supraoptic nucleus

Capillary network

Infundibulum

Axons carrying down
ADH, a neurosecretion

Anterior lobe (body)
of pituitary

Posterior lobe (body) of
pituitary

FIGURE 3.

Capillary network

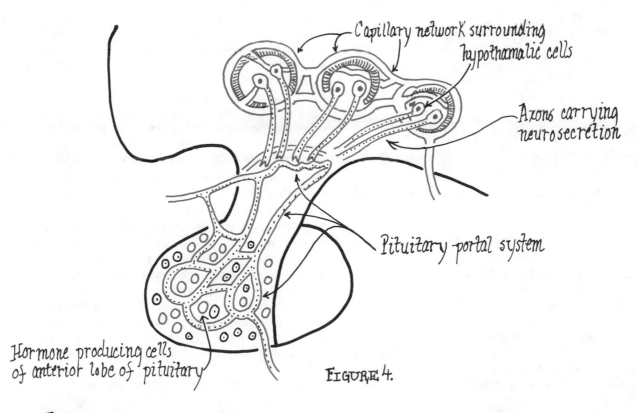

Capillary network surrounding
hypothalamic cells

Axons carrying
neurosecretion

Pituitary portal system

Hormone producing cells
of anterior lobe of pituitary

FIGURE 4.

PLATE 18-2.

WATER BALANCE

The hypothalamic mechanism for maintaining water balance is one of the most interesting regulatory mechanisms of the body. It is known that a hormone from the posterior pituitary body, called anti-diuretic hormone, or ADH, acts on the distal convoluted tubules of the kidney, causing resorption of water. If the amount of ADH produced is reduced, a pathological condition known as diabetes insipidus results. (With this disease the patient will urinate 18–20 liters of urine per day instead of the normal 1–2.) The regulatory mechanism in the production and release of ADH is a function of the supra-optic nucleus of the hypothalamus. The cells of this nucleus and possibly those of the paraventricular nucleus produce ADH, and this neurosecretion passes down the axons of the neurons, via the infundibulum, to reach the cells of the posterior pituitary (Figure 3), where the ADH is either stored or released into the capillary network.

If there is a reduction in the amount of water in the blood, the cells of the supra-optic nucleus, which are sensitive to such a change, will produce and release more ADH. This results in more water being resorbed by the kidney tubules and its conservation by the body. On the other hand, if there is a state of hydration, the cells of the supra-optic nucleus react by decreasing the production and release of ADH. This decrease in the production and release of ADH results in a decrease in the amount of water resorption by the kidneys and therefore a greater amount is urinated.

INFLUENCE OF THE HYPOTHALAMUS ON THE SECRETION OF HORMONES FROM THE ANTERIOR LOBE OF THE PITUITARY

There is much evidence that cells of the hypothalamus *can in part* influence the secretion of various hormones of the anterior lobe of the pituitary gland. The mechanism resembles that of water metabolism. Neurosecretory cells of the hypothalamus are very sensitive to the blood concentration of the various anterior lobe hormones. In response to a decrease, these neurons produce a neurosecretion that passes down the axons. However, the axons terminate in the region of the infundibulum and here the neurosecretion is "picked up" by a pituitary portal system (Figure 4). This carries the neurosecretion to the anterior lobe, where it stimulates the cells to produce the various hormones. One must not conclude that the hypothalamus is the only, or principal, regulator of hormones from the anterior lobe. There are other mechanisms, such as a direct feedback control, as well as mechanisms that are not yet clearly understood.

HYPOTHALAMIC DISCHARGE IN EMOTIONAL STATES

Various emotional states, such as anger or fear, result in physiological reactions. The hypothalamus is a center for the control and discharge of such reactions. For example, when one sees or hears something that evokes an angry reaction, the stimuli first reach various areas of the cerebral cortex, such as the visual or auditory centers, the memory centers, or the personality area of the frontal lobe, all of which are interconnected by association tracts. From the cerebral cortex, especially its frontal lobe, there is a discharge pathway to the hypothalamus. From the latter, the major descending pathway is the dorsal longitudinal fasciculus*, which arises from all the hypothalami, nuclei, and areas except the supra-optic and ventral median nucleus. This fasciculus leaves the hypothalamus and passes down the length of the brainstem, where it gives off branches to all the descending reticular nuclei, all the parasympathetic nuclei of cranial nerves III, VII, IX, and X, the respiratory and cardiac centers, and the motor nuclei of cranial nerves (Figure 2). From the reticular nuclei emerge the lateral and medial reticulospinal tracts, which descend the cord to supply the autonomic nervous system as well as the voluntary muscles. Thus, we see the complex interrelationship that exists between various parts of the brain, and one must proceed with great caution in applying new surgical or other techniques, e.g., lobotomies.

The hypothalamus is also involved in the olfactory reflex system (see Chapter 16). Finally, experimental work in animals has demonstrated that destruction of the ventral median nucleus produces animals with voracious — almost insatiable — appetites, while destruction of the lateral hypothalamic area produces animals that have no appetite. Clinically, we see that some patients who have tumors of the hypothalamus lose their appetites and become emaciated.

---

*A minor pathway is the mamillotegmental tract.

Chapter 19

THE CEREBRAL CORTEX

The cerebral cortex is most highly developed in humans. It is responsible for the qualities that distinguish humans from other animals: e.g., the ability to use the hand for skilled, intricate movements, a very high level of speech, symbolic thought, personality, and conscience. We know all this because if certain areas of the cortex are damaged these qualities are lost or greatly reduced.

In submammalian species the cerebral cortex is small and concerned almost exclusively with smell, which, as has already been described, is for them one of the most important sensations. The thalamus is the main sensory receptor area, while the basal ganglia and subthalamic nuclei serve as the motor discharge areas. Since fine, complicated voluntary movements don't exist in these lower forms, the cerebellum is primarily a center for equilibrium, which is a function of its flocculonodular lobe. As one ascends the evolutionary ladder, the cerebral cortex enlarges and takes on other functions. For example, the main sensory area is now localized in the postcentral gyrus and its former center, the thalamus, now becomes a center that relays the sensory impulses from the body to the cortex. With the appearance of the cerebral motor cortex, the basal ganglia in humans become areas of crude motor activity. Parallel with the development of this motor cortex there is a great development of the cerebellum as a coordination center for muscle activity, but the floccular nodulus remains the center for body equilibrium. In humans some functions, such as smell, decrease greatly in importance, although the complicated pathways remain — and drive medical students "up the walls."

With the increase in complexity and functions there is an increase in the number of neurons, and the area of cerebral cortex increases to such a degree that the cortex, in order to expand in the same volume area, is thrown into folds, giving us the characteristic appearance of gyri and sulci. (In lower forms, such as the rat, the surface of the cerebral cortex is smooth.) This principle is used by restaurant owners in high rent areas — instead of having straight counters, they make them convoluted, and thus squeeze in more customers.

As has been mentioned throughout this text, certain areas of the cortex have specific functions. The precentral gyrus, area 4, is concerned with initiating voluntary movements, while the postcentral gyrus, area 3,1,2, is the primary somatic sensory reception center. The occipital pole and the area on both sides of the calcarine fissure, area 17, form the primary visual receptor center. Areas 41 and 42, situated on the superior temporal gyrus, are the primary auditory reception center. Damage to any of these areas results in loss of function, such as paralysis, anesthesia, blindness, etc. In addition, area 8, lying anterior to area 6 in the frontal lobe (Figure 1), is concerned with voluntary conjugate movements of the eyes. The frontal poles and the areas surrounding them are the site of personality. A person who suffers injury to this area, say following a car accident, will probably undergo personality changes. The author remembers a case of a very friendly and pleasant social worker who suddenly and for no apparent reason became very argumentative and abusive, until her death a short while later. Autopsy revealed an expanding tumor in the frontal lobe that had caused both her death and the marked changes in character.

In the mid-1930s a Portuguese neurosurgeon, Moniz, introduced the procedure of cutting or removing parts of the frontal lobes — a lobotomy — as a means of treating severely psychotic patients. With hardly a murmur of dissent, this procedure was widely hailed (Moniz received the Nobel prize for it in 1949) and widely practiced. True, after the operation many of the patients were quieter and more docile, but they also lost all initiative, became indifferent to their surroundings, defecated and urinated in public, etc. Today this barbarous operation is thoroughly discredited; any

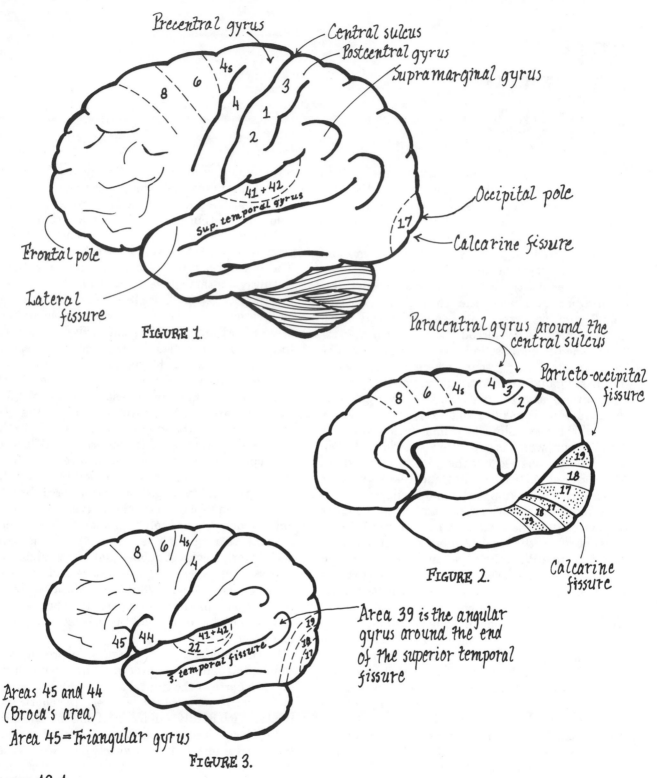

Precentral gyrus

Central sulcus
Postcentral gyrus
Supramarginal gyrus

8   6   4s   4   3   1   2

41 + 42
Sup. temporal gyrus

Occipital pole

17

Calcarine fissure

Frontal pole

Lateral fissure

FIGURE 1.

Paracentral gyrus around the central sulcus

Parieto-occipital fissure

8   6   4s   4   3   2

19
18
17
18   17
19

Calcarine fissure

FIGURE 2.

8   6   4s   4

45   44   41+42   22   s. temporal fissure

19
18
17

Area 39 is the angular gyrus around the end of the superior temporal fissure

Areas 45 and 44 (Broca's area)

Area 45 = Triangular gyrus

FIGURE 3.

PLATE 19-1.

surgeon contimplating it should take into account, among other things, the fact that Moniz was almost murdered by a former patient who was distraught over his new state. One can say that this was one case where the operation was a success but the surgeon nearly died!

Surrounding each of the primary cortical areas and closely allied with them are *associated areas*. Around the visual area, area 17, there are areas 18 and 19, which have several functions. First, they are concerned with "interpreting" the visual impulses that reach area 17. We see round, green objects in front of us and areas 18 and 19 interpret them as apples. This interpretation is called *gnosis*, from the Greek word meaning "to know." Area 19 is concerned with automatic following movements of the eyes, which occur when an object, such as a jet, suddenly comes into the visual field and the eyes "lock in" and follow it. Associated with area 4 is area 4s, the suppressor band, and area 6, which helps with voluntary movements. Area 22 is the auditory association area; if it is damaged on the dominant side, i.e., the left hemisphere in a right-handed person, then the patient can hear you speaking but can't understand what is being said. This condition is known as *word deafness*, or *auditory aphasia*, and is discussed in the following paragraph. (Aphasia is defined as the inability to understand or express the symbols connected with language, and there are two basic kinds: sensory and motor.)

SENSORY (RECEPTOR) APHASIA

If one traces the superior temporal sulcus to its posterior end, the gray matter surrounding this end is the *angular gyrus* — area 39 — of the parietal lobe (Figure 3). Damage to this area on the dominant cerebral hemisphere produces a condition known as *visual aphasia*, "word blindness," or *alexia*. In this condition the patient sees the printed words but he cannot read them and they are meaningless to him. This condition is equivalent to an occidental looking at Chinese writing; all he sees are curved lines and characters that have no specific meaning for him.

Area 22, surrounding the primary auditory reception areas (41 and 42), is the auditory reception area. If it is damaged, again on the dominant cerebral hemisphere, *auditory aphasia*, or "word deafness," results. The patient isn't deaf; he hears you speaking but he is unable to understand what you're saying. He experiences sound without any meaning; the same thing as when you hear a com-

pletely foreign language. *Wernicke's aphasia* is a condition of both auditory and visual aphasia.

MOTOR APHASIA

On the inferior frontal gyrus, in the triangular and opercular regions, are found areas 44 and 45, also known as *Broca's area* (Figure 3). If they are injured on the dominant hemisphere in an adult, they produce a condition in which the patient is unable to talk, even though the vocal muscles are not paralyzed. The patient knows what he wants to say, but all that comes out is garbled sound or one word repeated over and over again. One might say that the memory engrams connected with speech have been destroyed. If the damage occurs in childhood, the child can be taught to speak by utilizing the non-dominant cerebral hemisphere.

APRAXIA

Apraxia is the inability to carry out purposeful, learned, voluntary acts although there is no paralysis present. It also involves the association areas. When told to take out his keys and open the door, the patient pulls out a coin or comb and tries to put it into the keyhole. If the damage involves the loss of writing ability, it's known as *agraphia*.

AGNOSIA

Agnosia is the inability to recognize things although one sees them. A patient can walk down the street, see some broken glass in his way, and walk around it. However, when you ask him what it is he walked around, he doesn't know.

These conditions may sound strange, but many things concerning the cerebral cortex are so. As can readily be appreciated, the subject of aphasias and apraxias, as well as other cerebral conditions, such as epilepsy, are not as simple as has been presented here, but are very complex matters that have psychological aspects as well. Our "hard fact" knowledge is very restricted, and, since experiments can't be performed easily on the human cortex, what little information we have comes from pathological cases and autopsies. The reader who wishes to learn more about the telencephalon should consult *Correlative Anatomy of the Nervous System*, by Crosby, Humphrey, and Lauer, which has nearly 200 pages on the subject and over 1,300 references. There are also books available that are devoted to individual subject matters, such as epilepsy, EEG, etc.

Chapter 20

THE MENINGES

Brain tissue, having the consistency of a heavy pudding or custard, is the most delicate of all body tissues. For protection, this vital organ is located in a sealed bony chamber, the *skull*. To protect it further from the rough bone, blows and shocks to the head, etc., the brain is enveloped by three membranes, called the *meninges*. The outermost covering is the tough, thick *dura mater,* which is adherent to the inner surface of the bone (Figure 1). In fact, it forms the periosteal layer of the calvarium. Beneath the dura mater is the middle covering, the thin and filamentous *arachnoid*. The third and innermost layer is the very thin, delicate, and capillary-rich *pia mater,* which is attached directly to the brain and which dips down into the sulci and fissures (Figure 1).

Although the dura mater is closely applied to the inner bone surface, it can in certain instances separate from it, creating an area between the two known as the *epidural space* (see "Clinical Aspects" at the end of this chapter). Between the dura mater and the underlying arachnoid is a very narrow subdural space filled with a small amount of serous fluid that acts as a lubricant, preventing adhesion between the two membranes (Figure 1). Separating the arachnoid from the pia mater is a relatively large gap, the *subarachnoid space,* which is filled with cerebrospinal fluid (CSF) (Figure 1). This clear, lymph-like fluid fills the entire subarachnoid space and thus surrounds the brain with a protective "cushion" that absorbs shock waves to the head. As a further means of protection there are fibrous filaments known as the *arachnoid trabeculations,* which extend from the arachnoid to the pia and help "anchor the brain" in order to prevent it from excess movement in

cases of sudden acceleration or deceleration (Figure 1). In the fluid-filled subarachnoid space are situated the cerebral arteries and veins (Figure 1). The pia mater is so closely attached to the underlying brain that there is no space, potential or otherwise, between the two. In this manner the pia mater acts as a restraining agent that holds the brain tissue together and prevents it from separating.

The dura mater dips down into the median longitudinal fissure, and this dural fold, lying between the cerebral hemispheres, is called the *falx cerebri* (Figures 1 and 2). The dura also dips into the space between the cerebellum and the overlying occipital lobes. This is called the *tentorium cerebelli* (Figures 1 and 2) because it forms a tent-like covering over the cerebellum. Finally, the dura mater dips between the two cerebellar hemispheres to form the *falx cerebelli* (Figure 2).

CLINICAL ASPECTS

The middle meningeal artery doesn't supply the brain, but the dura of the middle cranial fossa. It lies between the dura mater and the skull, and in cases of severe trauma to the head, as in car accidents, jagged bone splinters can cut the artery. Then arterial blood, which is under high pressure, flows out rapidly between the dura and bone, forming a rapidly expanding pool that presses on the underlying brain. Unconsciousness soon follows and immediate surgical intervention is needed to prevent death. This condition and others are beautifully illustrated by Dr. Netter in the world-famous Ciba collection of atlases.

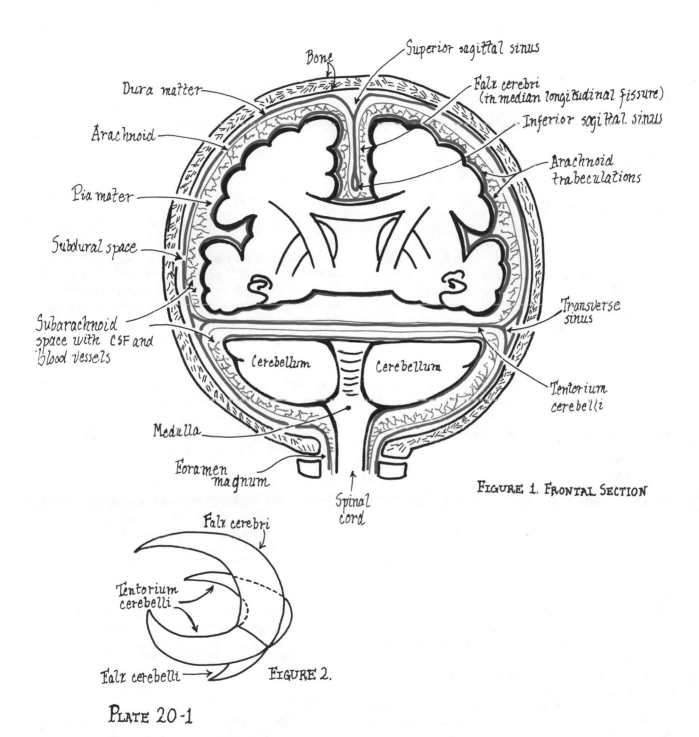

Bone

Superior sagittal sinus

Dura matter

Falx cerebri
(in median longitudinal fissure)

Arachnoid

Inferior sagittal sinus

Arachnoid
trabeculations

Pia mater

Subdural space

Subarachnoid
space with CSF and
blood vessels

Transverse
sinus

cerebellum

Cerebellum

Tentorium
cerebelli

Medulla

Foramen
magnum

Spinal
cord

FIGURE 1. FRONTAL SECTION

Falx cerebri

Tentorium
cerebelli

Falx cerebelli

FIGURE 2.

PLATE 20-1

Chapter 21

BLOOD SUPPLY TO THE BRAIN

As is mentioned in Chapter 1, nerve cells don't regenerate. They also need a constant, adequate supply of blood, and any interruption of it or injury to the vascular tree can quickly lead to irreparable, life-long damage or death. Since such injuries are commonly encountered in medical practice, knowledge and understanding of CNS vascularity is essential. Two pairs of arteries, the vertebrals and the internal carotids, are the only suppliers to the brain. The *vertebral arteries* enter the skull through the foramen magnum and pass along the ventral surface of the medulla (Figure 1). After giving off the *anterior* and *posterior spinal arteries* as well as the *posterior inferior cerebellar artery*, they join together to form the *basilar artery*, which passes up to the beginning of the pons, where it bifurcates into the *posterior cerebral arteries*. These sweep back to supply the posterior part of the cerebral hemispheres, especially the medial and basilar surfaces (Figures 1,2, and 3). In its course the basilar artery gives off the *anterior inferior cerebellar artery, pontine branches,* and the *superior cerebellar artery*.

The *internal carotid arteries* enter the skull through the foramen lacerum and lie adjacent to the lateral border of the optic chiasma (Figure 1). Here they bifurcate into the *anterior cerebral artery*, which passes forward into the medial longitudinal fissure and then sweeps back to the parieto-occipital fissure, thus supplying the medial surface of the hemisphere (Figures 1,2, and 3). The second branch of the internal carotid is the *middle cerebral artery*, which passes laterally between the temporal and frontal lobes. It emerges at the

lateral fissure and fans out to supply most of the lateral surface of the hemisphere (Figures 1 and 2). In its course between the temporal and frontal lobes, the middle cerebral artery gives off the very important *striate arteries,* which help supply the internal capsule, with its descending motor tracts (Figure 1). Because the striate arteries are the frequent site of cerebrovascular accidents (CVA), they are known as the "arteries of stroke."

The anterior cerebral arteries are connected to each other by the *anterior communicating artery.* There is also a posterior artery that links the middle cerebral artery with the posterior cerebral artery (Figure 1). Thus, at the base of the brain an anastomotic ring is formed between the vertebral and internal carotid arteries that is called the *Circle of Willis.* This is important clinically because if one of the arteries becomes occluded, the blood can pass around to reach the deprived area. In addition, the Circle of Willis is a frequent site for *aneurisms.* An aneurism forms when blood pressure at a weakening in the wall causes the artery to balloon out. An aneurism can press on adjacent structures, e.g., the optic chiasma, causing visual disturbances (Figure 1, and also refer to the chapter on visual pathways).

VENOUS DRAINAGE

Venous blood takes a roundabout circuit in its drainage to the neck. Most of the veins reach the surface of the brain and join larger veins. These cross the subarachnoid space and empty into large venous sinuses located within the dura

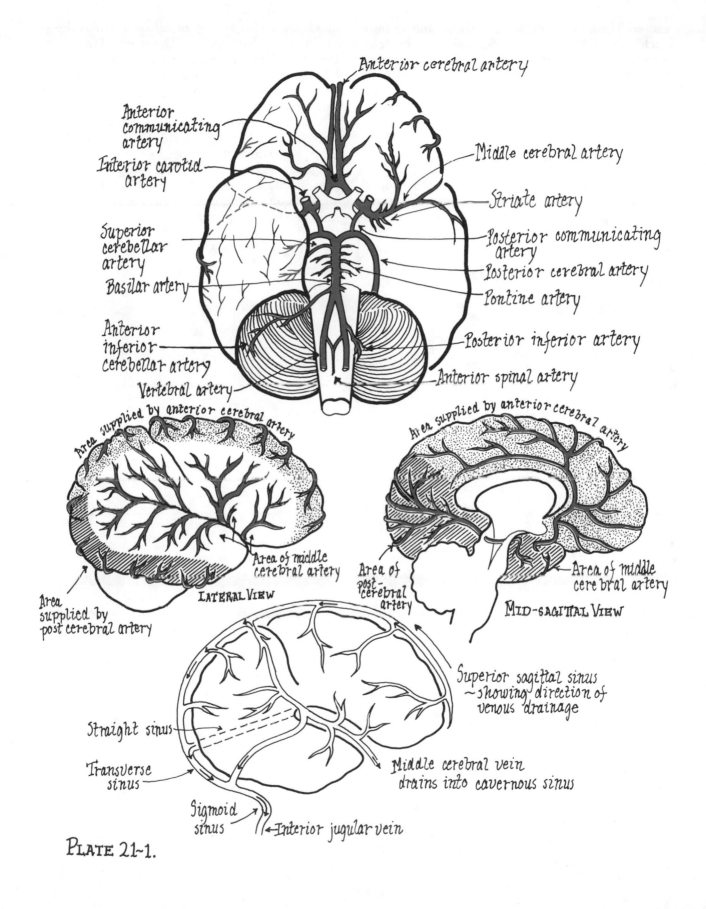

Anterior cerebral artery

Anterior communicating artery

Interior carotid artery

Superior cerebellar artery

Basilar artery

Anterior inferior cerebellar artery

Vertebral artery

Middle cerebral artery

Striate artery

Posterior communicating artery

Posterior cerebral artery

Pontine artery

Posterior inferior artery

Anterior spinal artery

Area supplied by anterior cerebral artery

Area of middle cerebral artery

LATERAL VIEW

Area supplied by post cerebral artery

Area supplied by anterior cerebral artery

Area of post- cerebral artery

Area of middle cerebral artery

MID-SAGITTAL VIEW

Superior sagittal sinus ~showing direction of venous drainage

Straight sinus

Transverse sinus

Sigmoid sinus

Middle cerebral vein drains into cavernous sinus

Interior jugular vein

PLATE 21-1.

mater. There is a confluence of these sinuses into each other: the superior sagittal and straight sinuses flow into the transverse, which continues into the sigmoid, which drains into the internal jugular vein of the neck. The middle cerebral vein flows into the cavernous sinus located at the base of the brain.

CLINICAL ASPECTS

If an artery becomes occluded by an embolism or through vasospasm, the area distal to the occlusion is deprived of its blood supply and the cells quickly die. This usually results in a stroke, the severity of which depends on the artery stopped and the site of occlusion, as well as other factors. Stroke, i.e., CVA, can also occur if an artery ruptures, and, if the hemorrhage is massive, death can occur very quickly.

Rupture of a vein occurs often in elderly people, frequently following a mild blow to the head. Since blood pressure is low in the veins, hemorrhage can be very slow and the symptoms may appear insidiously, several weeks after the trauma, which is often forgotten about because it was so mild and inconsequential.

Chapter 22

CEREBROSPINAL FLUID AND THE VENTRICULAR SYSTEM

Cerebrospinal fluid (CSF) is a clear fluid filling the entire subarachnoid space. It acts as a protective "liquid cushion" around the brain and spinal cord by absorbing shock waves from blows and falls. In addition, it is a valuable diagnostic aid: by means of a relatively simple procedure known as a spinal tap, the physician can obtain a fresh sample of the fluid, quickly examine it, and get an accurate picture of what is taking place within the skull and brain.

Deep inside the brain are a series of interconnecting chambers — the ventricular system — and it is here that CSF is produced. In each cerebral hemisphere there is a large space, the *lateral ventricle,* which is made up of an *anterior horn,* lying in the frontal lobe; the *body* or main part, lying in the frontal and parietal lobes; a *posterior horn,* in the occipital lobe; and an *inferior horn,* which sweeps down into the temporal lobe (Figures 1 and 2). In each lateral ventricle there is a delicate, lace-like structure, the *choroid plexus* (Figure 3), which is composed of pia mater enveloped by the thin membranous ependyma. Due to the hydrostatic pressure in the arteries, the CSF is extruded from the capillary-rich choroid plexus into the ventricular space; it is therefore similar to lymph. The accumulating CSF fills the lateral ventricles and then flows out of them via the interventricular *foramen of Munro* and into the third ventricle. This narrow, slit-like space lies in the midline between the walls of the right and left diencephalon (Figures 1 and 2; see also Figure 3 in the Atlas). The choroid plexus in the third ventricle also produces CSF, and all of the fluid flows into the narrow aqueduct of Sylvius, located in the midbrain (Figures 1 and 2; see also Figures 4, 11, and 12 in the Atlas). The aqueduct then empties into the fourth ventricle, found in the pons and medulla (Figures 1, 2, and 3, and Figure 4 in the Atlas). Here also is the choroid plexus, which produces CSF. In the thin roof of the fourth ventricle are three openings — the median *foramen of Magendie* and the two lateral *foramena of Luschka**. It is through these openings that the CSF leaves the ventricular system and flows into and completely fills the subarachnoid space around the brain and cord (Figures 2 and 3). In certain regions the arachnoid is situated far from the pia mater, and the enlarged subarachnoid space forms areas known as cisterns, e.g., the cisterna magna (Figure 3).

An important question is, since the CSF is constantly being produced, what happens to the excess fluid? In the area of the superior sagittal sinus, the arachnoid projects through small openings in the dura mater into the sinus. The accumulating CSF creates a pressure that forces the excess fluid out of the arachnoid projections and into the dural venous blood, which carries it away (Figures 3 and 4). In gross preparations these fine arachnoid projections resemble granules of sugar or salt, and are therefore called *arachnoid granulations.*

CLINICAL ASPECTS

Hydrocephalus

Most often in newborn infants, a blockage may form somewhere in the ventricular system. Consequently, the CSF is unable to flow out and accumulates in the ventricles, where it presses on the nervous tissue, causing a thinning out of the brain with a widening of the ventricles. Since the cranial bones of the baby have not yet fused, the expanding, fluid-filled brain separates the bones and the head enlarges tremendously. The exact cause of hydrocephalus is unknown, but it may be due to failure of the foramena or aqueducts to develop, or

---

**Note: M*agendie is *m*edian; *L*uschka is *l*ateral.

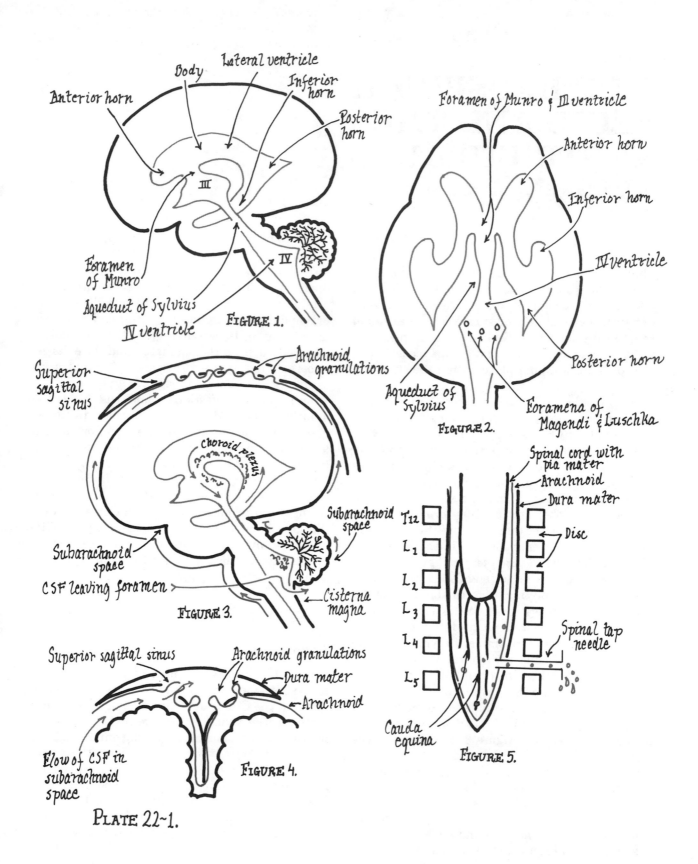

Anterior horn Body Lateral ventricle Inferior horn Posterior horn

III

IV

Foramen of Munro
Aqueduct of Sylvius
IV ventricle
FIGURE 1.

Foramen of Munro & III ventricle Anterior horn Inferior horn IV ventricle

Aqueduct of Sylvius Posterior horn Foramena of Magendi & Luschka
FIGURE 2.

Superior sagittal sinus Arachnoid granulations choroid plexus Subarachnoid space

Subarachnoid space CSF leaving foramen Cisterna magna
FIGURE 3.

Superior sagittal sinus Arachnoid granulations Dura mater Arachnoid

Flow of CSF in subarachnoid space FIGURE 4.

Spinal cord with pia mater Arachnoid Dura mater Disc Spinal tap needle

T12 L1 L2 L3 L4 L5

Cauda equina FIGURE 5.

PLATE 22~1.

they may become blocked following encephalitis (infection of the brain).

Spinal Tap

Since the spinal cord is shorter than the vertebral column, it generally ends at the level of the second or third lumbar vertebra (Figure 5). Therefore, the subarachnoid space below this level can be tapped with no danger of injuring the cord. After giving a local anesthetic, the doctor inserts a sterile hollow needle in between the fourth and fifth lumbar vertebra, punctures the dura mater, and enters the subarachnoid space filled with CSF. The hollow needle has a plunger, which is pulled out so that the CSF can then drip out. The physician measures the pressure of the intracranial CSF, which normally can reach 200 mm of water. In certain brain diseases the CSF pressure is greatly elevated. However, one must *never* attempt to reduce the pressure by letting out the CSF by means of a spinal tap, because the sudden downward flow of the released fluid pulls the brainstem into the foramen magnum, causing almost instantaneous death of the patient.

The spinal fluid obtained by spinal tap is examined for the presence of pus, blood, and bacteria and for the level of sugar, chloride, and protein.

In certain operations in which general anesthesia is contraindicated, local anesthetic fluid can be injected through the spinal tap needle into the epidural or subarachnoid space, producing what is known as a sacral or lumbar block. The anesthetist employs techniques that prevent the anesthetic fluid from flowing up the vertebral canal and silencing nerves to vital organs.

Appendix I

SPECIAL NEUROANATOMICAL GLOSSARY

WORD	DERIVATION	ILLUSTRATIVE EXAMPLE OR COGNATE
Alexia	*a,* "not" *lexia,* "to read"	Lexicon
Aqueduct	*aqua,* "water" *ductus,* "a leading"	Aquarium; Duke, "a leader of men"
Arachnoid	*arachne,* "spider" *edios,* "resemblance"	Arachnoid cells are web-like.
Arcuate	*arcus,* "a bow"	Arch; Archery
Astrocyte	*astron,* "star" *kytos,* "cell"	Astronomy
Brachium	"arm"	Embrace
Carotid	*karoo,* "to put to sleep"	Pressure on the carotid artery results in unconsciousness, as is well known in Judo.
Caudate	*cauda,* "a tail"	A caudate nucleus has a tail.
Cerebellum	*Cerebellum* is the diminutive of *cerebrum* ("brain"), and it means "little brain."	
Cerebrum	"brain"	Cerebration, "thinking"
Chiasma	The Greek letter chi — χ.	A chiasma is an arrangement in the form of a crossing.
Chorea	*choreia,* "dance"	People afflicted with Huntington's chorea exhibit characteristic ("dancing") movements. Choreography
Cistern	"a well"	
Claustrum	"enclosure"	Claustrophobia; Closet
Coronary	*corona,* "crown" or "garland" ALSO — The *corona radiata* is a fan-shaped ("radiating") fiber mass on the cerebral cortex.	The coronary arteries encircle the heart. Coronation
Corpus callosum	*corpus,* "body" *callosum,* "hard"	Callus; Corporation
Cortex	"bark"	The cerebral cortex covers the cerebral hemisphere, much as bark covers the trunk of a tree.
Cuneate	*cuneatus,* "made wedge-shaped"	The cuneiform writing of ancient Babylon had wedge-shaped characters.
Decussation	The Roman numeral X is called *deca.*	A decussation is a crossing.
Dendrite	"branching figure" or "bush"	Rhododendron

continued

WORD	DERIVATION	ILLUSTRATIVE EXAMPLE OR COGNATE
Dentate	*dens,* "tooth"	Dentist
	dentatus, "tooth-shaped"	
Dura mater	*dura,* "hard"	Durable; Alma mater
	mater, "mother"	
Epi-	"upon, over, above"	
Fasciculus	"a bundle" (of rods or fibers)	The symbol of the Italian *Fascists* was the Roman bundle of rods, the *fascis* seen on old Mercury Head dimes.
Fornix	"arch"	In ancient Rome the prostitutes hung around the supporting arches of the viaducts. A man visiting the area was engaged in fornication.
Genu	"bend"	Genuflect, i.e., bend (bow) before royalty
Glia	"glue"	Glial cells "hold together" the neurons.
Glossal	*glossa,* "tongue"	Glossary
Gracilis	"slender"	
Gyrus	*gyros,* "ring, circle"	Gyrate; Gyroscope
Hippocampus	*hippo,* "horse"	In cross-section the hippocampus resembles a seahorse. Hippodrome
	campus, "sea"	
Hypo-	"under, below"	A hypodermic goes under the skin (*dermis*).
Insula	"island"	Insulin is produced by the islands of Langerhans. Insulation
Internuncial	*inter,* "between"	Announce; Papal nuncio
	nuncio, "messenger"	
Lemniscus	"ribbon, band"	
Lentiform	"lens-shaped"	*Lens* is the Latin word for lentil, the "lens-shaped" vegetable of the bean family.
Limbic	*limbus,* "border" or "edge"	Limbo is the area bordering on Hell.
Lingula	"little tongue"	Linguist; Language
Lumbar	*lumbus,* "loin" or "flank"	Lumbago
Mamillary	"breast shaped"	Mammary; mammals
Mesencephalon	*meso,* "middle"	Mezzanine
	encephalon, "in the brain"	
Oligodendroglia	*oligo,* "few"	Oligarchy, "a few who rule"
	dendro, "branching figure" or "bush"	
	glia, "glue"	
Pallidus	"pale"	The pallidus is pale in comparison to the neighboring putamen.
Peduncle	"foot, limb, stalk"	Pedal; Pedestrian
Pia mater	*pia,* "soft, delicate"	Pianissimo
	mater, "mother"	
Pineal	*pinea,* "pine cone"	The pineal body is conical.
Pons	"bridge"	Pontoon
Ramus	"branch"	Ramifications
Rectus	"straight"	Rectify
Reticular	*reticulum,* "small net"	A reticle is the network of lines in a telescopic sight; a lady's reticule is a small net bag.
Rhinencephalon	*rhino,* "nose"	Rhinocerous
	encephalon, "in the brain"	
Rubro	"red"	Ruby

continued

WORD	DERIVATION	ILLUSTRATIVE EXAMPLE OR COGNATE
Sacral	"holy, sacred"	The sacral bone was believed to resist decomposition and thus serve as the basis for resurrection.
Sagittal	*sagitta,* "arrow"	Sagittarius is the Archer of the zodiac.
Sella turcica	"Turkish saddle" — which it resembles	
Septum	"a partition"	Separate
Substantia nigra	"black substance"	Nigeria; Negro
Tapetum	"carpet"	Tapestry
Tectum	"roof"	Architecture
Temporal	*tempus,* "time"	The temporal area gives evidence of the passage of time, i.e., the hair turns gray.
Tentorium	"tent"	
Tubercle	"a swelling" or "rounded projection"	Tubers (potatoes); Protuberance
Vagus	"wandering"	The vagus nerve extends into the thorax and abdomen. Vagabond; vagrant
Velum	"covering"	Veil
Ventricle	*ventrus,* "chamber, cavity, hollow, stomach"	A ventriloquist "speaks from the stomach."
Vermis	"worm" — which it resembles	

Appendix **II**

ATLAS OF
THE BRAIN

ATLAS. PLATE I. LATERAL VIEW OF THE BRAIN.

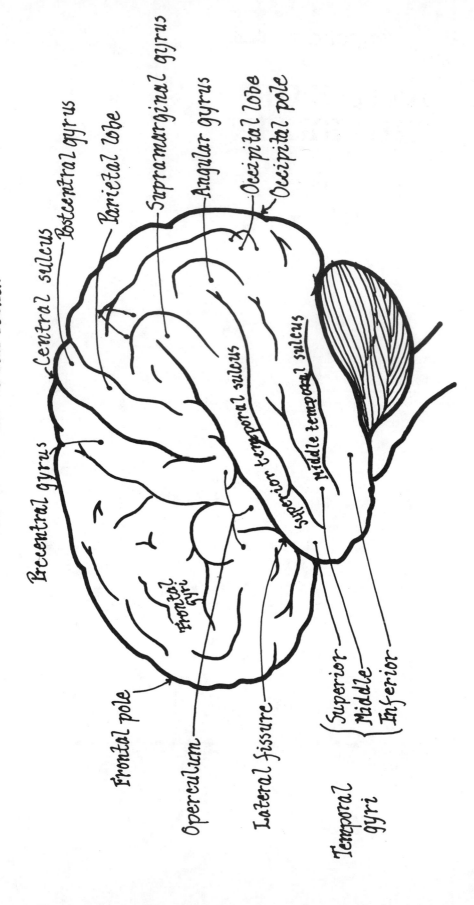

Precentral gyrus

Central sulcus

Postcentral gyrus

Parietal lobe

Supramarginal gyrus

Angular gyrus

Occipital lobe

Occipital pole

Frontal gyri

Superior temporal sulcus

Middle temporal sulcus

Frontal pole

Operculum

Lateral fissure

Temporal gyri { Superior Middle Inferior

ATLAS. PLATE II. BASAL VIEW OF THE BRAIN.*

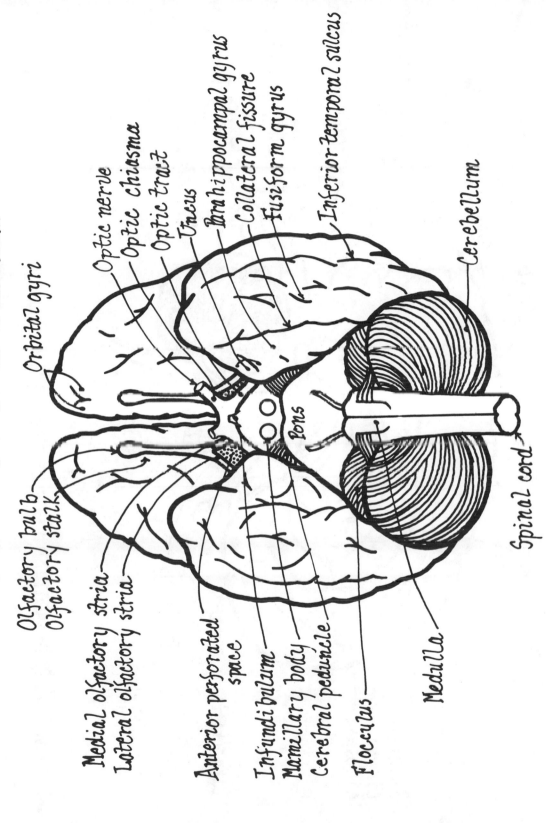

Olfactory bulb
Olfactory stalk

Orbital gyri

Optic nerve
Optic chiasma
Optic tract

Uncus

Parahippocampal gyrus
Collateral fissure
Fusiform gyrus

Inferior temporal sulcus

Cerebellum

Medial olfactory stria
Lateral olfactory stria

Anterior perforated space

Infundibulum
Mamillary body
Cerebral peduncle

Flocculus

Pons

Medulla

Spinal cord

* For a more detailed view of the brainstem with the cranial nerves, see PLATE VIII of this atlas.

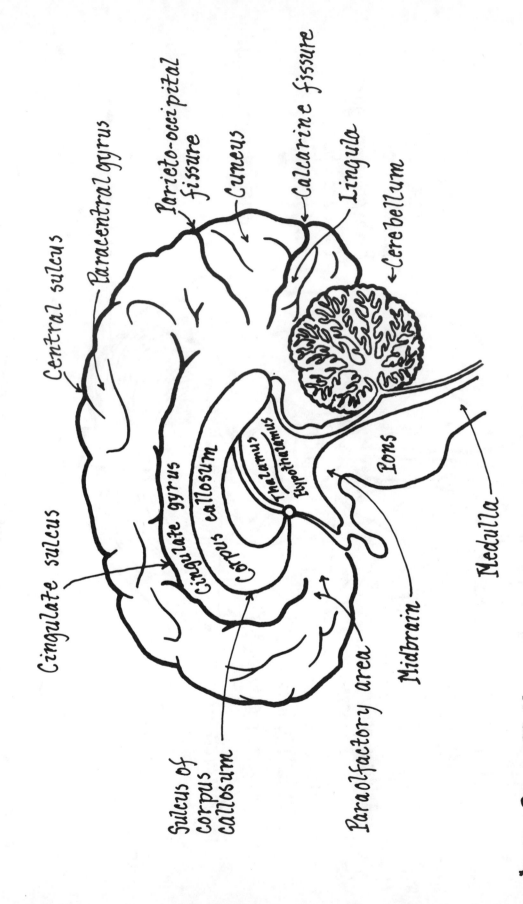

Central sulcus

Paracentral gyrus

Parieto-occipital fissure

Cuneus

Calcarine fissure

Lingula

Cerebellum

Cingulate sulcus

Cingulate gyrus

Corpus callosum

Thalamus

Hypothalamus

Pons

Sulcus of corpus callosum

Paraolfactory area

Midbrain

Medulla

ATLAS. PLATE III. MID-SAGITTAL VIEW OF THE BRAIN.

ATLAS. PLATE IV. ENLARGED MID-SAGITTAL VIEW OF THE BRAIN.

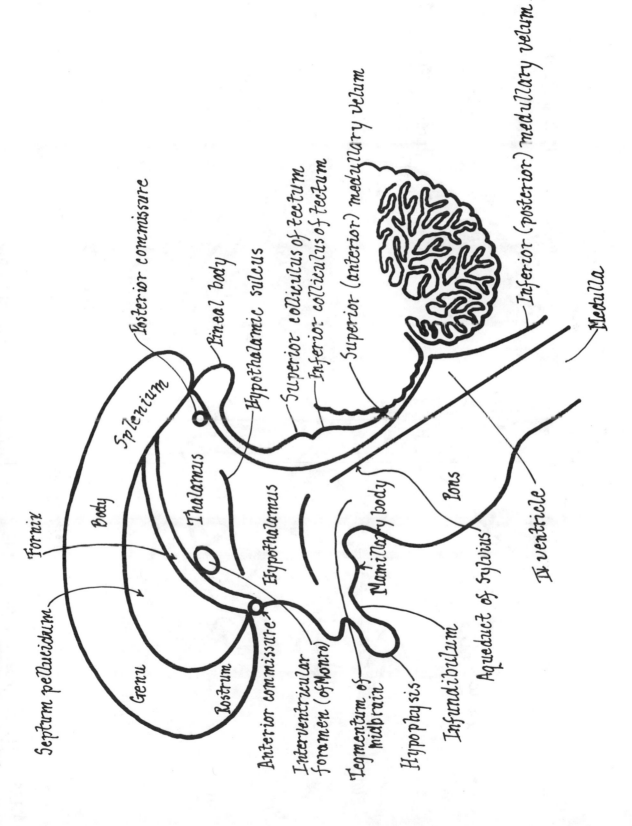

Septum pellucidum

Fornix

Body

Genu

Rostrum

Splenium

Posterior commissure

Pineal body

Hypothalamic sulcus

Superior colliculus of tectum

Inferior colliculus of tectum

Superior (anterior) medullary velum

Inferior (posterior) medullary velum

Medulla

Thalamus

Hypothalamus

Anterior commissure

Interventricular foramen (of Monro)

Tegmentum of midbrain

Hypophysis

Infundibulum

Mamillary body

Aqueduct of Sylvius

Pons

IV ventricle

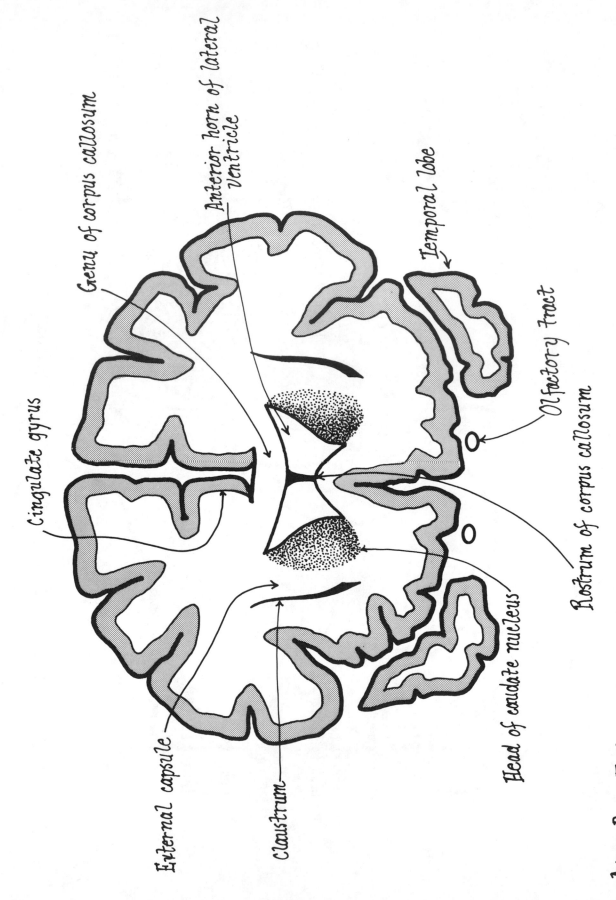

ATLAS. PLATE V. CROSS-SECTION OF THE BRAIN, ANTERIOR TO THE ANTERIOR COMMISSURE.

Genu of corpus callosum

Anterior horn of lateral ventricle

Temporal lobe

Cingulate gyrus

Olfactory Tract

Rostrum of corpus callosum

External capsule

Head of caudate nucleus

Claustrum

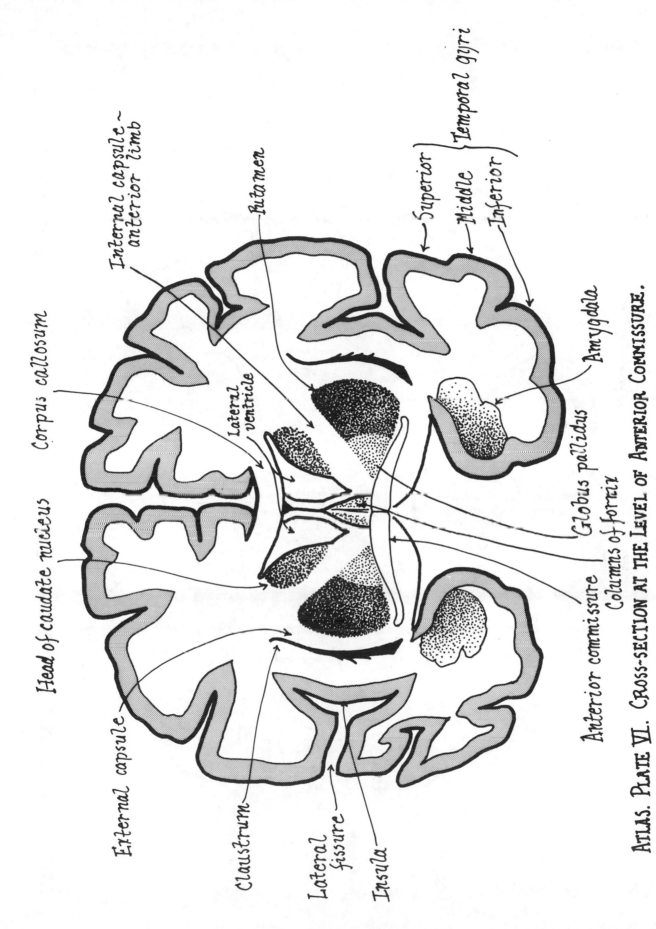

Internal capsule ~ anterior limb

Putamen

Superior ⎫
Middle ⎬ Temporal gyri
Inferior ⎭

Corpus callosum

Head of caudate nucleus

Lateral ventricle

Amygdala

Globus pallidus

External capsule ~

Claustrum

Lateral fissure

Insula

Anterior commissure
Columns of fornix

ATLAS. PLATE VI. CROSS-SECTION AT THE LEVEL OF ANTERIOR COMMISSURE.

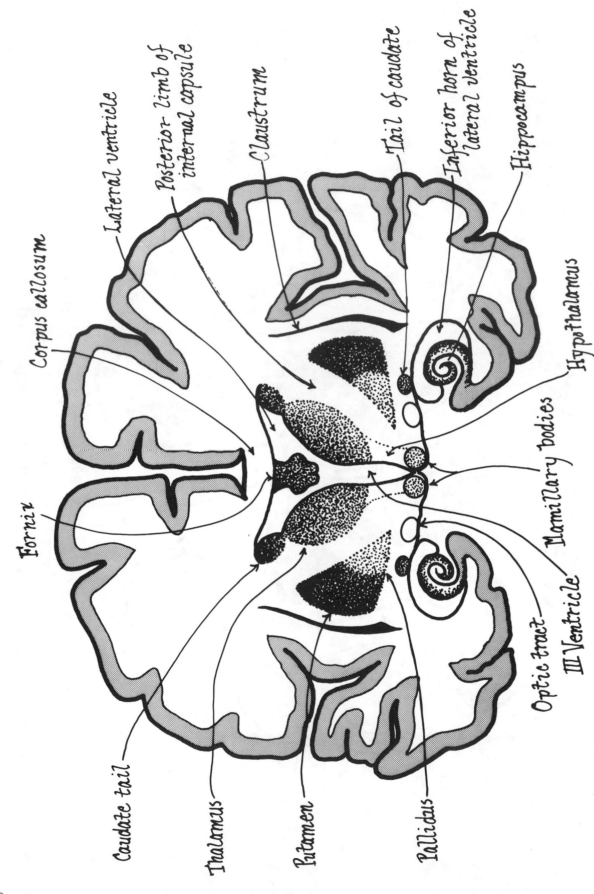

Corpus callosum

Lateral ventricle

Posterior limb of internal capsule

Claustrum

Tail of caudate

Inferior horn of lateral ventricle

Hippocampus

Fornix

Hypothalamus

Caudate tail

Thalamus

Putamen

Optic tract

Mamillary bodies

III Ventricle

Pallidus

ATLAS. PLATE VII. CROSS-SECTION OF THE BRAIN AT THE LEVEL OF THE MAMILLARY BODIES.

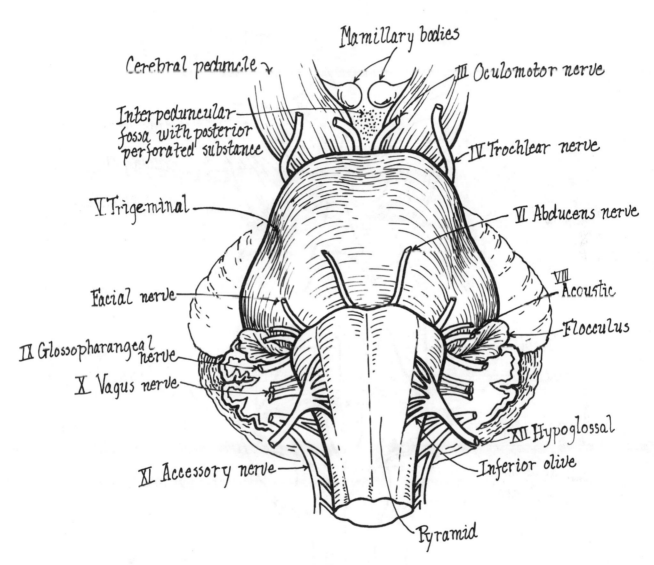

Mamillary bodies

Cerebral peduncle

III Oculomotor nerve

Interpeduncular fossa with posterior perforated substance

IV Trochlear nerve

V Trigeminal

VI Abducens nerve

VIII Acoustic

Facial nerve

Flocculus

IX Glossopharangeal nerve

X Vagus nerve

XII Hypoglossal

Inferior olive

XI Accessory nerve

Pyramid

ATLAS. PLATE VIII. VENTRAL VIEW OF THE BRAINSTEM.

89

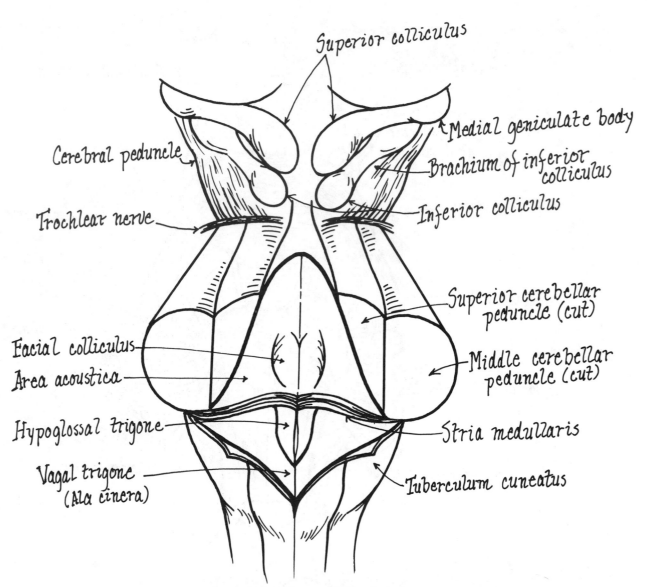

Superior colliculus

Cerebral peduncle

Trochlear nerve

Facial colliculus
Area acoustica

Hypoglossal trigone

Vagal trigone
(Ala cinera)

Medial geniculate body
Brachium of inferior colliculus
Inferior colliculus

Superior cerebellar peduncle (cut)

Middle cerebellar peduncle (cut)

Stria medullaris

Tuberculum cuneatus

ATLAS. PLATE IX. DORSAL VIEW OF THE BRAINSTEM.

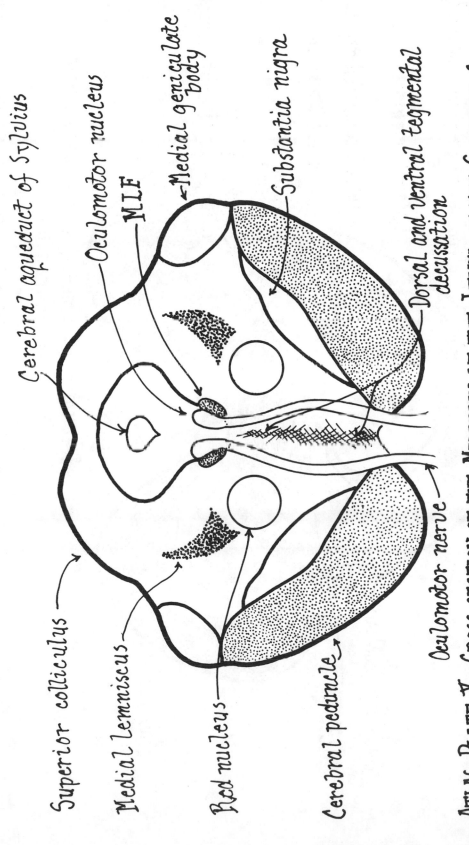

Cerebral aqueduct of Sylvius

Oculomotor nucleus

MLF

Medial geniculate body

Substantia nigra

Dorsal and ventral tegmental decussation

Superior colliculus

Medial lemniscus

Red nucleus

Cerebral peduncle

Oculomotor nerve

ATLAS. PLATE X. CROSS-SECTION OF THE MIDBRAIN AT THE LEVEL OF THE SUPERIOR COLLICULUS.

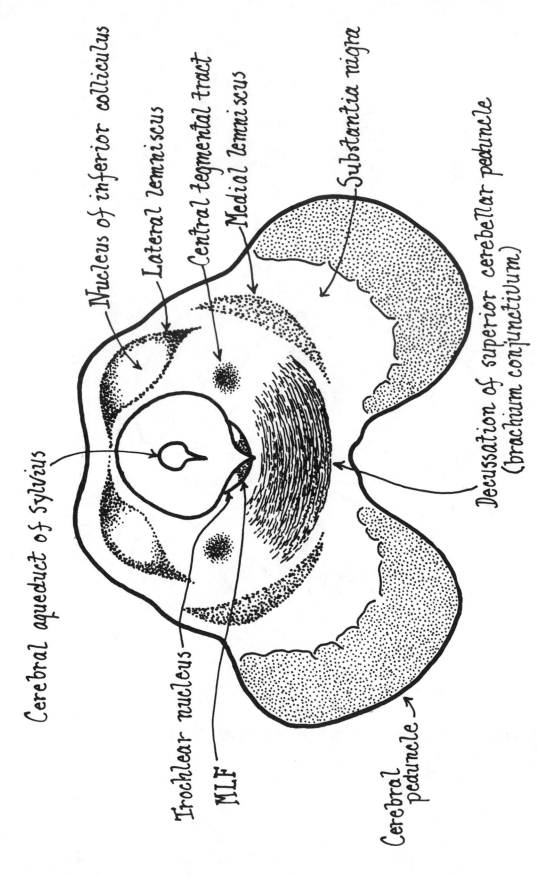

Cerebral aqueduct of Sylvius

Nucleus of inferior colliculus

Lateral lemniscus

Central tegmental tract

Medial lemniscus

Substantia nigra

Decussation of superior cerebellar peduncle (brachium conjunctivum)

Trochlear nucleus

MLF

Cerebral peduncle →

ATLAS. PLATE XI. CROSS-SECTION OF THE MIDBRAIN AT THE LEVEL OF THE INFERIOR COLLICULUS.

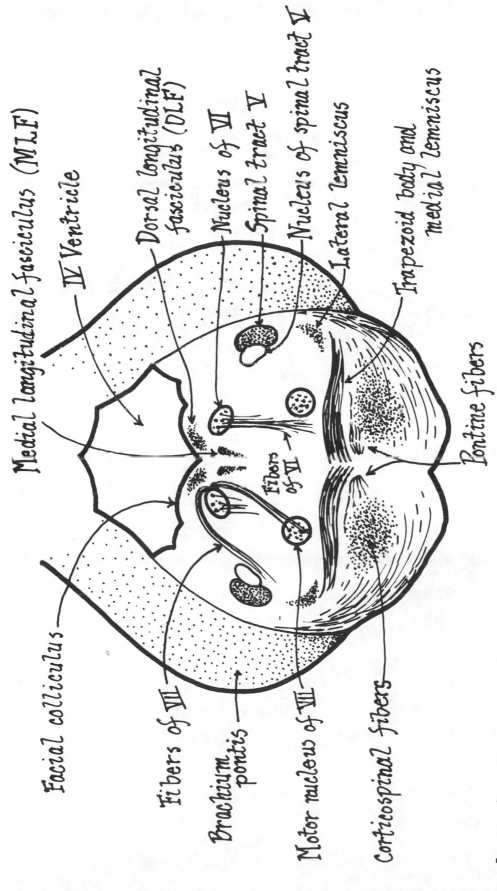

Medial longitudinal fasciculus (MLF)

IV Ventricle

Dorsal longitudinal fasciculus (DLF)

Nucleus of VI

Spinal tract V

Nucleus of spinal tract V

Lateral lemniscus

Trapezoid body and medial lemniscus

Pontine fibers

Fibers of VI

Facial colliculus

Fibers of VII

Brachium pontis

Motor nucleus of VII

Corticospinal fibers

ATLAS. PLATE XII. CROSS-SECTION OF THE PONS AT THE FACIAL COLLICULUS.

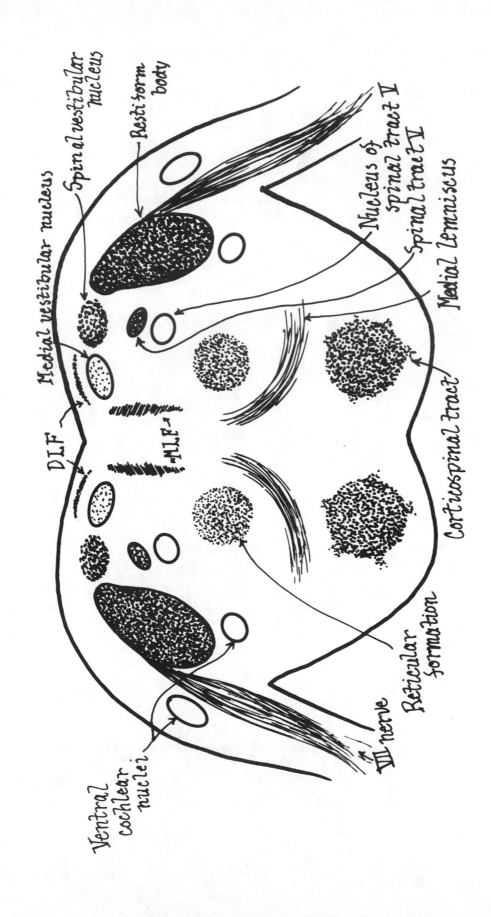

Spinal vestibular nucleus

Restiform body

Nucleus of spinal tract V

Spinal tract V

Medial Lemniscus

Medial vestibular nucleus

DLF

MLF

Corticospinal tract

Reticular formation

VII nerve

Ventral cochlear nuclei

ATLAS. PLATE XIII. CROSS-SECTION OF LOWER PONS.

94

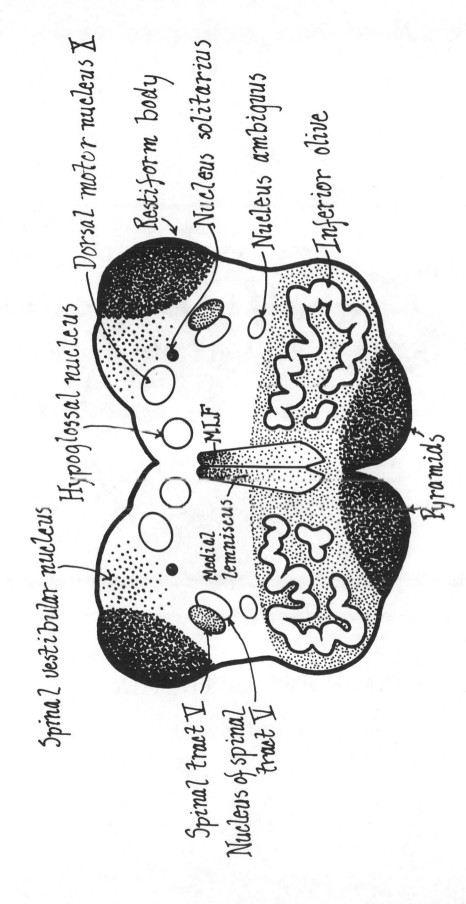

Spinal vestibular nucleus

Hypoglossal nucleus

Dorsal motor nucleus X

Restiform body

Nucleus solitarius

Nucleus ambiguus

Inferior olive

MLF

Medial lemniscus

Spinal tract V

Nucleus of spinal tract V

Pyramids

ATLAS. PLATE XIV. SECTION THROUGH UPPER MEDULLA.

95

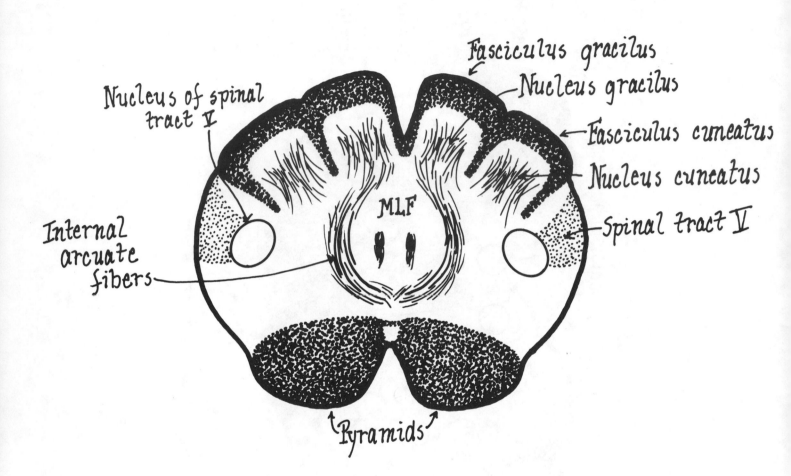

Nucleus of spinal tract Ⅴ

Internal arcuate fibers

Fasciculus gracilus

Nucleus gracilus

Fasciculus cuneatus

Nucleus cuneatus

Spinal tract Ⅴ

MLF

Pyramids

ATLAS. PLATE ⅩⅤ. SECTION THROUGH LOWER MEDULLA.

Appendix III

SAMPLE EXAMINATION QUESTIONS

1. Which of the following tracts or pathways is completely uncrossed in its entire course?
   - a. Pain and temperature from the face
   - b. Proprioception from the body
   - c. Corticospinal
   - d. Dorsal spinocerebellar
   - e. Vestibular pathways

2. What condition results if the right optic nerve is cut?
   - a. Left homonymous hemianopsia
   - b. Bitemporal hemianopsia
   - c. Right homonymous hemianopsia
   - d. Binasal hemianopsia
   - e. None of the above

3. Which of the following is not true concerning the hypothalamus?
   - a. Concerned with temperature regulation
   - b. Has a hunger center
   - c. Is concerned with equilibrium
   - d. Influences pituitary secretions
   - e. Has areas concerned with emotional reactions

4. Which of the following statements concerning the neuron is not true?
   - a. Very sensitive to oxygen deprivation
   - b. If the axon is cut the cell body will always die
   - c. Myelin is laid down by the sheath of Schwann
   - d. Nissl bodies are found in the cytoplasm of the cell body
   - e. Mature neurons don't undergo mitosis

5. Which of the following tracts doesn't synapse on the final common pathway?
   - a. Rubrospinal tract
   - b. Corticospinal tract
   - c. Spinothalamic tract
   - d. Vestibulospinal tract
   - e. All of the above

6. Which of the following is not a sign of cerebellar injury?
   - a. Uncoordinated movements
   - b. Dizziness
   - c. Athetosis
   - d. Falling
   - e. Intention tremor

In the following three questions match the tract with the peduncle in which it runs:
7. Corticopontocerebellar tract
8. Dentorubrothalamic tract
9. Vestibulocerebellar tract
   - a. Superior cerebellar peduncle
   - b. Middle cerebellar peduncle
   - c. Inferior cerebellar peduncle

10.   Obstruction of the left anterior cerebral artery is likely to cause defective movement of the:
  a.   Right lower limb
  b.   Right upper limb
  c.   Muscles of the face on the left side
  d.   Muscles of the face on the right side
  e.   Left lower limb

11.   With respect to the sub-cortical motor areas, i.e., basal ganglia, etc., all of the following statements are true except:
  a.   Damage to them can result in pill-rolling tremor
  b.   They aren't connected to the cerebral cortex
  c.   They are part of the extrapyramidal system
  d.   They are connected with the red nucleus
  e.   They are connected with the thalamus

12.   A patient exhibits bitemporal hemianopsia. In which of the following areas is the lesion most likely to be?
  a.   Lateral geniculate body
  b.   Midline of the optic chiasma
  c.   Optic radiations
  d.   Visual cortex
  e.   Optic tract

13.   Which of the following doesn't synapse in the thalamus?
  a.   Pain and temperature from the face
  b.   Fibers from the dentate nucleus
  c.   Proprioception from the body
  d.   Auditory fibers
  e.   Pressure and touch from the face

14.   A patient suffers from an upper neuron paralysis that affects his arm. The lesion can be in all of the following areas except:
  a.   Motor cortex
  b.   Internal capsule
  c.   Cerebral peduncles
  d.   Tegmentum of the midbrain
  e.   Pyramid
  f.   Lateral white column of the spinal cord

15.   If the dorsal spinal root is cut in the sacral region, which of the following would show Wallerian degeneration in the cervical area of the cord?
  a.   Spinothalamic tract
  b.   Fascilulus cuneatus
  c.   Ventral spinocerebellar tract
  d.   Lateral corticospinal tract
  e.   Fasiculus gracilis

16.   The cell bodies of the preganglionic parasympathetic fibers that innervate the descending colon are situated in the:
  a.   Dorsal motor nucleus of the vagus
  b.   Nucleus ambiguus
  c.   Lateral gray column of the spinal cord in the 10–12 thoracic segments
  d.   Inferior mesenteric ganglion
  e.   Lateral gray column of the spinal cord in the 2–4 sacral segments

17.   A patient has total deafness in the left ear. In which of the following areas is the lesion most likely to be?
  a.   Left superior temporal gyrus
  b.   Right and left cochlear nuclei
  c.   Left auditory nerve
  d.   Left lateral lemniscus
  e.   Right and left inferior collilculi

18.   Examination reveals that a patient doesn't sweat in the area supplied by thoracic spinal nerves T_1–T_2. A lesion in which area *won't* give rise to this condition?
    a.   Sympathetic trunk
    b.   Intermediate lateral gray column of the spinal cord
    c.   Ventral roots of the spinal cord
    d.   White rami communicantes
    e.   Doral roots of spinal nerve
    f.   Gray rami communicantes

In the following three questions three common reflexes are listed. Match them with the correct cranial nerves that are involved in the reflex arc.

19.   Corneal reflex
20.   Horizontal nystagmus
21.   Gag reflex
    a.   optic - facial
    b.   vestibular - facial
    c.   glossopharyngeal - vagus
    d.   vestibular - oculomotor and abducens
    e.   trigeminal - facial
    f.   trigeminal - vagus

Answer the following questions by indicating the letter of the statement that correctly applies.
    a.   If both statements are true and there is a causal relationship between the two.
    b.   If both statements are true but there is no causal relationship between the two.
    c.   If the first statement is true but the second is false.
    d.   If the first statement is false and the second is true.
    e.   If both statements are false.

22.   Most of the spinocerebellar fibers enter the cerebellum on the ipsilateral side and therefore injury to the right inferior cerebellar peduncle results in a person falling to the right side.

23.   Damage to the genu of the left internal capsule results in a paralysis of the entire right side of the face because the corticobulbar fibers are located in the genu of the internal capsule.

24.   If the right thalamus is damaged then the patient will lose all somatic sensations on the left side of the body and face because these fibers all eventually cross over to the opposite side from which they entered the cord and brainstem.

ANSWERS

1. d	6. c	11. b	16. e	21. c
2. e	7. b	12. b	17. c	22. a
3. c	8. a	13. d	18. e	23. d
4. b	9. c	14. d	19. e	24. e
5. c	10. a	15. e	20. d	

Index

macrophages, 1
macula, 53
mamillary bodies, 5, 64, 82, 84, 87, 88
mamillothalamic tract, 58, 59
mamillotegmental tract, 58, 59, 60, 61
medial geniculate body, 6, 50, 51, 52, 90
medial lemniscus, 13, 14, 90, 91, 92, 93
    injury to, 13–15
medial longitudinal fasciculus, 31, 32, 90, 91, 92–93
median longitudinal fissure, 4, 5, 54
median nuclei, 64
medulla oblongata, 5, 6, 7, 14, 20, 24, 30, 83
medulla
    lower, section through, 93
    upper, section through, 93
medullary velum
    inferior (posterior), 84
    superior (anterior), 84
Ménière's disease, 31
meninges, 70–71
mesencephalic nucleus, 17
mesencephalon, structure and function, 6
mesenteric ganglion
    inferior, 39
    superior, 39
microglia, 1
midbrain, 6, 7, 14, 24, 27, 36, 51, 83
    cross-section at level of inferior colliculus, 90
    cross-section at level of superior colliculus, 90
MLF, see medial longitudinal fasciculus
monoplegia, 22
motor cortex, 23
motor decussation, 20
motor neuron, 1, 2
    see also lower motor neuron; upper motor neuron
mucous gland, 39
myelin, 1, 2
myelinization, 1, 3

neoplasms, 3
nervi erigentes, 40
nerve(s)
    repair of injury to, 3
    see also cranial nerve(s); spinal nerves
nerve impulse, transmittal of, 1
neuroblastomas, 3
neurolemma, 1
neuron, 1
    motor, or efferent, 1, 2
    sensory, or afferent, 1, 2, 9
    structure, 1
    types of, 2

see also lower motor neuron; motor neuron; upper motor neuron
Nissl granules, 1, 2
nodes of Ranvier, 1, 2
nodose ganglion, 44
nucleolus, 1, 2
nucleus(i), 2, 23
nucleus ambiguus, 23, 44, 93
nucleus cuneatus, 14, 93
nucleus gracilis, 14, 93
nucleus of Perla, 56
nucleus solitarius, 44, 46, 48, 93
nystagmus, 31, 35

occipital lobe, 4, 5, 82
occipital pole, 7, 53, 54, 67, 68, 82
oculomotor nucleus, 7, 40, 55, 90
oculomotor nerve, 6, 7, 23–25, 32, 40, 41, 44, 45, 46, 88, 90
olfactory bulb, 58, 82
olfactory nerve, 4, 5, 43, 44
olfactory stalk, 82
olfactory stria, 82
olfactory tract, 85
oligodendroglia, 1
olivary nucleus, superior, 50, 51
olivocerebellar tract, 33
operculum, 82
optic chiasma, 53, 54, 82
optic nerve, 4, 5, 43, 44, 54, 82
optic radiation, 53, 54
optic tracts, 4, 53, 54, 82, 87
orbital gyri, 4, 5, 82
otic ganglion, 40, 46

pain
    phantom limb, 10
    receptors, 8
    referred, 10
pain and temperature pathway
    from face, 16
    somatic, 8–10
paracentral gyrus, 7, 68, 83
parahippocampal gyrus, 82
paralysis, 19, 21–22
paraolfactory area, 57, 58, 83
paraplegia, 22
parasympathetic nervous system, 38, 41–42
paraventral nucleus, 64
paravertebral chain ganglia, 38
parietal lobe, 4, 5, 82
parieto-occipital fissure, 4, 5, 7, 54, 68, 83
Parkinsonism, 26–28, 35
parotid gland, 40
pelvic splanchnic nerves, 40
perforated area, 88
    anterior, 57, 58, 82
peripheral nerve(s), 2, 12
peripheral nervous system, parts of, 4

petrosal ganglion, 46
phagocytes, 1
phantom limb, 10
pia mater, 70, 71
pineal body, 6, 84
pituitary gland, 53, 54, 65
pituitary, hormone secretion, 66
pons, 5, 7, 17, 24, 30, 51, 82, 83
    cross-section at facial colliculus, 91
    lower, cross-section of, 92
    structure, 6
pontine nuclei, 36
postcentral gyrus, 5, 8, 9, 12, 13, 14, 16, 17, 67, 68, 82
    injury to, 13–15
posterior commissure, 55, 56, 84
posterior limb, 7
posterior ventral nucleus of the thalamus, 9
postganglionic fiber, 41
precentral gyrus, 4, 5, 20, 23, 24, 27, 67, 68, 82
preganglionic fiber, 38
preoptic nucleus, 64
pressure receptors, 11
pretectal nucleus, 55, 56
projection fibers, 6
proprioception, 13
    pathway
        from face, 16–17
        somatic, 13–15
proprioceptive fibers, 33
pterygopalatine ganglion, 48
ptosis, 45
pupillary dilator muscle, 39
Purkinje cell of cerebellum, 2
putamen, 7, 26, 27, 86, 87
pyramid(s), 20, 88, 93
pyramidal system, 26
pyramidal tract, 19, 20
    suppressor part, 21

quadriplegia, 22

receptor, 2
receptor in dermis, 12
red nucleus, 6, 7, 26, 27, 35, 37, 90
referred pain, 10
reflex, 8
    blink, 18
restiform body, 6, 34, 36, 92, 93
reticular area, 37
reticular formation, 26, 92
    ascending, 60–62
    descending, 60, 61
reticular nuclei, 60, 61, 63, 64
reticular system, 60–62
reticulospinal tract, 26, 27, 35, 37, 60, 61, 64
reticulocerebellar tract, 33
retina, 53